PRINCIPLES OF

OCULAR IMAGING

Praise for *Principles of Ocular Imaging*

What a timely, practical, and informative textbook. A truly comprehensive resource on a multitude of ocular imaging modalities. A must-read for all health care professionals involved in vision care.

—Eduardo C. Alfonso, MD
Professor and Chairman
Kathleen and Stanley J. Glaser Chair in Ophthalmology
Bascom Palmer Eye Institute

Principles of Ocular Imaging is a beautiful, handy visual guide to all types of ocular imaging—from the traditional to the most cutting-edge. Drs. Gologorsky and Rosen have done an incredible job. A must-have for all ophthalmologists!

—Amy Schefler, MD
Associate Professor of Clinical Ophthalmology
Weill Cornell Medicine
Houston Methodist Hospital and University of Texas Health Science Center of Houston

This is an excellent textbook that provides insight about the various evolving imaging modalities for everyone from trainees to practicing ophthalmologists.

—Ajay Kuriyan, MD, MS
Assistant Professor
Mid Atlantic Retina
Wills Eye Hospital
Thomas Jefferson University

This beautifully illustrated 256-page text provides the reader with concise paragraphs of clinical wisdom followed by selected timely references. The topics range from Oculoplastics to Neuro-Ophthalmology and Glaucoma. My favorite sections were Retina and Cornea, which showcase the latest technologies. Easy reading and excellent images make this book useful for all clinicians.

—Harry W. Flynn, MD
Professor of Ophthalmology
J. Donald M. Gass Chair in Ophthalmology
Bascom Palmer Eye Institute

The emergence of ocular imaging technologies over the last two decades has changed the landscape of eye care. No longer are advanced technologies only found in specialty practices or academic university settings, but instead are being utilized in all kinds of practices across the country by both optometrists and ophthalmologists—ultimately allowing us to take better care of our patients.

The textbook Principles of Ocular Imaging by Daniel Gologorsky, MD and Richard B. Rosen, MD is a comprehensive guide to 22 imaging technologies that are widely used in eye care. It not only includes a detailed review of each imaging technology but provides the most clinically relevant aspects as well as great examples highlighting each of the technologies. This will become one of those must-have textbooks for every practice and will become the foundation for understanding imaging in eye care.

—Mark T. Dunbar, OD
Director of Optometric Services
Bascom Palmer Eye Institute

PRINCIPLES OF
OCULAR
IMAGING

Editors

Daniel Gologorsky, MD, MBA

Chief of Ophthalmology
Broward Health Medical Center
Fort Lauderdale, Florida
Medical Director
Miami Eye and Retina
Miami Beach, Florida

Richard B. Rosen, MD, ScD(hon), FACS, FASRS, FARVO, CRA

Belinda B. and Gerald G. Pierce Distinguished Chair of Ophthalmology
Deputy Chair of Clinical Affairs and Vice Chair of Ophthalmology Research
Surgeon Director and Retina, System Chief
New York Eye and Ear Infirmary of Mount Sinai
Professor of Ophthalmology
Icahn School of Medicine at Mount Sinai
New York, New York
Honorary Professor of Applied Optics
School of Physical Sciences
University of Kent
Canterbury, United Kingdom

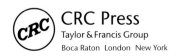

CRC Press
Taylor & Francis Group
Boca Raton London New York

CRC Press is an imprint of the
Taylor & Francis Group, an **informa** business

First published 2021 by SLACK Incorporated

Published 2024 by CRC Press
2385 NW Executive Center Drive, Suite 320, Boca Raton FL 33431

and by CRC Press
4 Park Square, Milton Park, Abingdon, Oxon, OX14 4RN

CRC Press is an imprint of Taylor & Francis Group, LLC

Cover Artist: Katherine Christie

Library of Congress Cataloging-in-Publication Data

Names: Gologorsky, Daniel, editor. | Rosen, Richard B., editor.
Title: Principles of ocular imaging / [edited by] Daniel Gologorsky, Richard B. Rosen.
Description: Thorofare, NJ : SLACK Incorporated, [2021] | Includes
   bibliographical references and index.
Identifiers: LCCN 2020010669 | ISBN 9781630915995 (hardcover)
Subjects: MESH: Eye--anatomy & histology | Eye--diagnostic imaging | Atlas
Classification: LCC QP475 | NLM WW 17 | DDC 612.8/4--dc23
LC record available at https://lccn.loc.gov/2020010669

ISBN: 9781630915995 (hbk)
ISBN: 9781003525929 (ebk)

DOI: 10.1201/9781003525929

DEDICATION

To my parents, whose humility, grace, and integrity are matched by their relentless spirit, love of learning, and prodigious erudition. To my siblings, whose encouragement, love, and guidance have been bulwarks of support. And to my wonderful wife and children, who have imbued my life with absolute joy and endowed it with a deeper sense of purpose.

"Our eyes register the light of dead stars."
—*André Schwarz-Bart* in ***The Last of the Just***

We ophthalmologists obsess over all matters related to light and vision. This book is dedicated to the shimmering lights, those curious dreamers and thinkers whose vision was extinguished by the atrocities of the 20th century.

—*Daniel Gologorsky, MD, MBA*

To my inspiring teachers, Frank Gollan, Morton Rosenthal, Donald Gass, Lawton Smith, Joseph Walsh, Thomas Muldoon, and my invigorating students, residents, and fellows for inspiring me to look beyond the obvious. To my role-model parents who allowed me to pursue my dreams from childhood and retain my child into adulthood. To my captivating wife, three amazing sons, and two precious grandsons who have filled my life with joy and made it all make sense.

—*Richard B. Rosen, MD*

"Discovery consists of seeing what everyone else has seen and thinking what no one else has thought."
—*Albert Szent-Gyorgyi*

"You can observe a lot, just by watching."
—*Yogi Berra*

"There's a difference between looking and seeing."
—*Thomas Muldoon*

CONTENTS

Dedication..*vii*
About the Editors...*xiii*
Contributing Authors..*xv*
Preface...*xvii*
Foreword...*xix*
Introduction...*xxi*

Section I   **Oculoplastics** **1**
            Section Editor: *Wendy W. Lee, MD, MS*

Chapter 1   External Photography 3
            Alexandra E. Levitt, MD, MPH; Apostolos Anagnostopoulos, MD; and
            Wendy W. Lee, MD, MS

Chapter 2   Ptosis Visual Fields 11
            Alexandra E. Levitt, MD, MPH; Apostolos Anagnostopoulos, MD;
            Ann Q. Tran, MD; and Wendy W. Lee, MD, MS

Chapter 3   Slit Lamp Photography 17
            Ashwinee Ragam, MD

Chapter 4   Orbital Ultrasonography 27
            Ying Chen, MD; Andrew J. Rong, MD; Amy Huang, BS; John Hinkle, MD;
            Nimesh Patel, MD; and Wendy W. Lee, MD, MS

Section II **Cornea and Refractive** **35**
            Section Editors: *Ashwinee Ragam, MD and Oriel Spierer, MD*

Chapter 5   Corneal Topography 37
            Ashwinee Ragam, MD

Chapter 6   Confocal Microscopy 45
            Ashwinee Ragam, MD

Chapter 7   Anterior Segment Optical Coherence Tomography 51
            C. Maxwell Medert, MD; Hasenin Al-khersan, MD; and Ann Q. Tran, MD

Chapter 8   Ultrasound Biomicroscopy 57
            Ashwinee Ragam, MD

Chapter 9   Biometry for Intraocular Lens Calculations 61
            Ashwinee Ragam, MD

Section III   **Retina** **69**
Section Editors: *Daniel Gologorsky, MD, MBA and Richard B. Rosen, MD*

Chapter 10   Fundus Photography 71
Daniel Gologorsky, MD, MBA

Chapter 11   Fluorescein Angiography 81
Daniel Gologorsky, MD, MBA

Chapter 12   Indocyanine Green Angiography 93
Daniel Gologorsky, MD, MBA

Chapter 13   Fundus Autofluorescence 99
Hasenin Al-khersan, MD and Ann Q. Tran, MD

Chapter 14   Optical Coherence Tomography in Retina 109
Daniel Gologorsky, MD, MBA

Chapter 15   Optical Coherence Tomography Angiography 119
Chris Y. Wu, MD and Richard B. Rosen, MD

Chapter 16   Adaptive Optics 135
Chris Y. Wu, MD and Richard B. Rosen, MD

Chapter 17   Microperimetry 149
Hasenin Al-khersan, MD; Thomas Lazzarini, MD; and Ann Q. Tran, MD

Chapter 18   Retinal Ultrasonography 153
Daniel Gologorsky, MD, MBA and Yale Fisher, MD

Chapter 19   Electrophysiology of Vision 161
Alessandra Bertolucci, MD

Section IV   **Glaucoma** **173**
Section Editor: *Stephen Moster, MD*

Chapter 20   Visual Fields in Glaucoma 175
Stephen Moster, MD; Cindy X. Zheng, MD; and Michael M. Lin, MD

Chapter 21   Optical Coherence Tomography in Glaucoma 185
Michael M. Lin, MD; Cindy X. Zheng, MD; and Stephen Moster, MD

Section V   **Neuro-Ophthalmology** **199**
             Section Editor: *Wendy W. Lee, MD, MS*

Chapter 22   Computed Tomography and Magnetic Resonance Imaging............... 201
             Michelle W. Latting, MD; John W. Latting, MD; Sheikh Faheem, MD; and
             Wendy W. Lee, MD, MS

Bibliography 213
Financial Disclosures... 223
Index 225

ABOUT THE EDITORS

Daniel Gologorsky, MD, MBA is an ophthalmologist and vitreoretinal specialist trained at the Bascom Palmer Eye Institute and the New York Eye and Ear Infirmary. He completed his undergraduate studies at Cornell University, and obtained his MD and MBA degrees from Dartmouth Medical School and the Tuck School of Business at Dartmouth, respectively. He has authored more than 50 peer-reviewed publications and textbook chapters, and has lectured extensively at national and international ophthalmological conferences. Dr. Gologorsky serves as the Chief of Ophthalmology at Broward Health Medical Center in Fort Lauderdale, Florida.

Dr. Gologorsky enjoys teaching and is an avid history aficionado, with special interests in classical Rome and World War II. He is an entrepreneurship enthusiast, especially in the biotech space. He resides in Miami Beach with his wife, an endocrinologist, and their family.

Richard B. Rosen, MD is a vitreoretinal surgeon and medical retina consultant at the New York Eye and Ear Infirmary, where he serves as Deputy Chair of Clinical Affairs, Vice Chairman and Director of Ophthalmology Research, as well as Surgeon Director, System Chair of Retina and Retina Fellowship Director. Dr. Rosen holds the Belinda B. and Gerald G. Pierce Distinguished Chair of Ophthalmology and is Professor of Ophthalmology at the Icahn School of Medicine at Mount Sinai. He is President of the New York Eye and Ear Infirmary Ophthalmology Associates PC. He is also Honorary Professor in Applied Optics at the University of Kent in Canterbury, United Kingdom, where he was awarded an Honorary Doctorate in Medical Physics. His received his bachelor's degree in psychology and anthropology at the University of Michigan and his MD from the University of Miami School of Medicine. He also did graduate work in psychophysics in the Laboratory of Neuro-magnetism at New York University, and worked for several years as a professional photographer in New York City, with an interest in ophthalmic/scientific photography.

Dr. Rosen's research interests include new treatments for macular degeneration and diabetic retinopathy, innovations in diagnostic retinal imaging, and vitreoretinal surgical instrumentation. Dr. Rosen has authored two books, numerous book chapters, and more than 150 articles in peer-reviewed journals. He has served on the executive board of the American Society of Ocular Trauma, the editorial boards of *Retinal Physician* and *Ophthalmic Surgery, Lasers and Imaging Retina*, and multiple committees of the American Academy of Ophthalmology and the Association for Research in Vision and Ophthalmology.

CONTRIBUTING AUTHORS

Hasenin Al-khersan, MD (Chapters 7, 13, and 17)
Bascom Palmer Eye Institute
Miami, Florida

Apostolos Anagnostopoulos, MD (Chapters 1 and 2)
Bascom Palmer Eye Institute
University of Miami Miller School of
   Medicine
Miami, Florida

Alessandra Bertolucci, MD (Chapter 19)
New York Eye and Ear Infirmary of
   Mount Sinai
New York, New York

Ying Chen, MD (Chapter 4)
Bascom Palmer Eye Institute
Miami, Florida

Sheikh Faheem, MD (Chapter 22)
Assistant Professor
Carle Illinois College of Medicine
Carle Foundation Hospital
Urbana, Illinois

Yale Fisher, MD (Chapter 18)
Vitreous Retina Macula Consultants
New York, New York
Bascom Palmer Eye Institute
Miami, Florida

John Hinkle, MD (Chapter 4)
Wills Eye Hospital
Philadelphia, Pennsylvania

Amy Huang, BS (Chapter 4)
University of Colorado
Aurora, Colorado

John W. Latting, MD (Chapter 22)
Associate Physician
Radiology
The Permanente Medical Group
Modesto, California

Michelle W. Latting, MD (Chapter 22)
Associate Physician
Oculoplastic Surgery
The Permanente Medical Group
Stockton, California

Thomas Lazzarini, MD (Chapter 17)
Bascom Palmer Eye Institute
University of Miami Miller School of
   Medicine
Miami, Florida

Wendy W. Lee, MD, MS (Sections I and V and Chapters 1, 2, 4, and 22)
Professor of Clinical Ophthalmology and
   Dermatology
Oculofacial Plastic & Reconstructive Surgery,
   Orbit and Oncology
Bascom Palmer Eye Institute
University of Miami Miller School of
   Medicine
Miami, Florida

Alexandra E. Levitt, MD, MPH (Chapters 1 and 2)
Bascom Palmer Eye Institute
Miami, Florida

Michael M. Lin, MD (Chapters 20 and 21)
Massachusetts Eye and Ear
Boston, Massachusetts

C. Maxwell Medert, MD (Chapter 7)
Bascom Palmer Eye Institute
Miami, Florida

Stephen Moster, MD (Section IV and Chapters 20 and 21)
Temple University
Philadelphia, Pennsylvania

Nimesh Patel, MD (Chapter 4)
Bascom Palmer Eye Institute
Miami, Florida

Ashwinee Ragam, MD (Section II and Chapters 3, 5, 6, 8, and 9)
New York Eye and Ear Infirmary of Mount Sinai
New York, New York

Andrew J. Rong, MD (Chapter 4)
Bascom Palmer Eye Institute
University of Miami Miller School of Medicine
Miami, Florida

Oriel Spierer, MD (Section II)
Sackler Faculty of Medicine
Tel Aviv University
Tel Aviv, Israel

Ann Q. Tran, MD (Chapters 2, 7, 13, and 17)
Bascom Palmer Eye Institute
Miami, Florida
Manhattan Eye Ear Nose and Throat Hospital
Northwell Health
New York, New York

Demetrios G. Vavvas, MD, PhD (Foreword)
Monte J. Wallace Ophthalmology Chair in Retina
Ophthalmology
Harvard Medical School
Massachusetts Eye and Ear Infirmary and Massachusetts General Hospital

Chris Y. Wu, MD (Chapters 15 and 16)
Shiley Eye Institute
University of California San Diego
La Jolla, California

Cindy X. Zheng, MD (Chapters 20 and 21)
Clinical Assistant Professor of Ophthalmology
Eye Physicians
Voorhees, New Jersey
Wills Eye Hospital
Philadelphia, Pennsylvania

PREFACE

Boris Pasternak once quipped, "It is not the object described that matters, but the light that falls on it." Our understanding of disease is fundamentally limited by our perception of it. We are fortunate to live in an era in which various imaging modalities can empower our diagnostic agility. A discerning clinician will understand the limitations of and the differences between the image and the device taking the image; an object and our perception of it; and disease and artifact. It takes acumen to recognize when to order a test and, perhaps more importantly, when not to.

Ophthalmology residency at the Bascom Palmer Eye Institute came with a steep learning curve. Although as medical students and interns we had significant exposure to CT scans, MRIs, and EKGs, there was virtually no exposure to ocular imaging modalities such as optical coherence tomography, fluorescein angiography, or visual fields. During my first week of ophthalmology training, I checked out a dozen textbooks on ophthalmic imaging from my residency's library, desperate for clinical competency in a milieu in which such familiarity is often assumed.

I learned that ophthalmology is inextricably intertwined with imaging; today it is impossible to be a cataract surgeon without biometry, or to properly manage retinal diseases without optical coherence tomography. It was at this point in my residency that I conceived of the need for this book: a comprehensive guide to all ophthalmic imaging for the eye specialist wishing to know of and understand the latest imaging developments.

For this first edition we prioritized 22 distinct imaging modalities, most of which are unique to ophthalmology. We organized these topics (comprising the individual chapters of this book) by anatomy (anterior to posterior) and subspecialty, and exerted considerable effort to provide a concise but thorough technical background, with many highly illustrative examples demonstrating how to apply the principles of that modality in a real-life clinical context.

I am thankful to all the contributors who participated in this project, and am especially grateful to Dr. Richard Rosen for inspiring his students to love and appreciate ophthalmic imaging.

—*Daniel Gologorsky, MD, MBA*

FOREWORD

The Greek word for eye (ὀφθαλμός) is a composite of the verb to see (ὁράω-ὁρῶ-ὄπωπα) and the noun for chamber (θαλμός-θάλαμος). Thus, the eye is defined as an instrument needed for visualization. It is only fitting that this instrument we use to see should benefit the most from instruments of visualization.

Advances in understanding of the anatomy and function of the eye began in antiquity from careful observations using the naked eye. Using dissection, Aristotle described the three main layers of the eye. Rufus added the conjunctiva layer, and Galen made contributions to the anterior and posterior chambers, and added some basic understanding of the curvature of the cornea and lens.

From medieval Islamic times, some imprecisions were propagated, such as the location of the lens in the center of the eye. This concept remained until the more modern times of the 18th century ushered in a renaissance of the field, with the development of new imaging instruments.

In the late 1700s and 1800s the epicenter of eye studies moved to Europe, with such notables as J. Freke, oculist Baron de Wenzel, Sir Duke Elder, Ernst Abbe (of Zeiss, working on microscopes), and Hermann von Helmholtz (who invented the ophthalmoscope in 1851). Soon thereafter, the first description of photographing the retina by Jackman and Webster was published in 1886.

In 1911 the Swede Allvar Gullstrand both declined (for Physics) and accepted (for Physiology and Medicine) the Nobel Prize for his work and contribution to the understanding of the eye as a refractive organ. He remains the only ophthalmologist to win a Nobel Prize for work in Ophthalmology. During that same year, he presented in Heidelberg his work on the slit lamp prototype. It would take until 1916, with the advancement in bulb technology by Walther Nernst (another Nobel laureate), before the slit lamp was truly realized. The slit lamp, combined with the binocular microscope developed by Czapski of Zeiss Factories, has since become the universal diagnostic tool for eye specialists for the last 100+ years!

The 20th and 21st centuries have witnessed an explosion in imaging, from the simple technique of indentation gonioscopy by Alexios Trantas, to fluorescein angiography introduced by medical students Novotny and Alvis of the University of Indiana in the 1960s, onward to the invention of optical coherence tomography by the team of James Fujimoto at the Massachusetts Institute of Technology in 1990, a technology destined for a future Nobel Prize.

Ophthalmology is at the forefront of medical imaging and ophthalmologists remain the only physicians who have almost complete mastery of imaging within their own specialty. This is unlike other medical fields, where the imaging expert (radiologist) and the clinician do not share the complete knowledge of the organ and the imaging modalities.

The explosion of imaging techniques available to today's modern ophthalmologist is both a blessing and a burden. How should one best use these tools efficiently and appropriately? How can one avoid being fooled by artifacts? Where should the beginner go to gain an understanding of this bounty of knowledge? This book by Gologorsky and Rosen was constructed as a concise but comprehensive introduction to ocular imaging, designed to facilitate immediate understanding and appropriate use. Ocular imaging is both an advanced science and a beautiful art. It is what inspired many of us to enter this magnificent field. Hopefully this book will do the same for the reader!

—Demetrios G. Vavvas, MD, PhD

INTRODUCTION

Imaging is an extension of our senses, an outreach of our abilities to see and hear and explore our environment. Examination of the eye, our most far-reaching facility, has expanded rapidly over the past few decades, beyond simple confrontation with magnification, to complex strategies designed to reveal blood circulation, detect discrepancies in form and function, and inconsistencies at the cellular level. Imaging allows us to reach into the eye with delicate probes of light and sound to interrogate the vitality of responses and judge normalcy.

With the growing complexity of new imaging tools, clinicians are now called upon to make quantitative as well as qualitative assessments of features and facilities that were previously unreachable. Successful deployment of this growing arsenal of sensory enhancements compels us to develop new ways of thinking about the familiar in order to take advantage of the new revelations presented.

The first real advance over face-to-face examination occurred in 1851 with Herman Helmholtz's introduction of the direct ophthalmoscope. This ushered in an era of explosive observation and innovation with rapid improvements upon his seminal device. What followed were a flurry of depictions of this new world inside the globe, advancing from observation and artists' renderings to the magic of photographic emulsions.

Henry Noyes of the New York Eye Infirmary is credited with taking the first photograph of a living fundus, a rabbit, in 1862. It was not until 23 years later that Lucien Howe presented the first human retinal image in 1885, followed by Dr. Theodore Jackman and Dr. Joseph Webster, who were first to publish a sample fundus image in 1886. Steady improvements in ophthalmoscopes and photography allowed Dr. Friedrich Dimmer and Dr. Arnold Pilate to publish a major atlas using a device manufactured by Zeiss in 1927.

Electroretinography, which was first revealed in amphibian retina in 1865 by Alarick Holmgren and in human retina by James Dewar in 1877, awaited introduction of the contact-lens electrode in 1941 by Lorin Riggs before it reached the clinic. Interpretation floundered until the work of Ragnar Granit in the 1960s.

In 1911, Allvar Gullstrand advanced the field of corneal imaging and access to the anterior segment of the eye with the introduction of the slit lamp with its multidimensional illumination features. Continued improvements have made it the mainstay of the ophthalmologist's examination lane.

In 1956, Henry Mundt and William Hughes demonstrated the first diagnostic application of ultrasound to the eye. Early work focused on A-mode scanning, which eventually found application in biometry for intraocular lenses. B-mode scanning, currently a mainstay of clinical diagnosis, was first introduced in a handheld probe by Nathanial Bronson and Frank Turner. Subsequently, it has evolved to encompass higher frequencies for high-resolution scans of the anterior segment and three dimensions for volumetric reconstructions.

A major leap forward in functional imaging occurred with the introduction of fluorescein angiography by medical students Harold Novotny and David Alvis in 1961. This helped open the field of medical retina led by ophthalmologist, pathologist, and observer extraordinaire Donald Gass and his Miami team, which included neuro-ophthalmologist Nobel David and ophthalmic photographer Johnny Justice. Other leaders in the photography field, including Don Wong, helped to codify the profession of ophthalmic photography with the foundation of the Ophthalmic Photographers' Society.

With the expansion of video technology and digital imaging, Rob Webb, Oleg Pomeranzeff, and George Hughes introduced the scanning laser ophthalmoscope (SLO) in 1980 at the Schepens Eye Institute. This jettisoned the field beyond the limits of optical images to reconstructions of point-by-point acquired scans and enabled functional testing at exact retinal foci, so-called fundus-based perimetry or microperimetry.

Within a decade, the next major advance was the introduction of optical coherence tomography (OCT) in 1990 by James Fujimoto and David Huang. This resulted in a seismic shift by revealing details along the cross-sectional perspective akin to a histopathology viewpoint. Adrian Podoleanu and David Jackson further empowered this new technology with the melding of the SLO to the OCT in 1997. They introduced en-face OCT, which would eventually serve as the platform for OCT angiography when it was made practical 15 years later by Yali Jai, David Huang, and Ruikang Wang.

Also in 1997, David Williams, Don Miller, Michael Morris, and Junzhong Liang pioneered the use of adaptive optics, originally developed for astronomy, to visualize individual photoreceptors and open the door to single-cell imaging of the living retina.

Today clinicians enjoy a rich smorgasbord of tools with which to study patients' visual systems from the surface of the cornea to the tip of the visual cortex. Many of the laborious components of the physical examination have been supplanted by micron-resolution tools that diagnose and treat a vast array of ocular disease.

In this volume the contributors have tried to provide the most clinically relevant aspects of each of today's mainstream imaging tools in an easily accessible format for a quick study. Many next-generation advances wait in the wings as scientists, engineers, and researchers conspire to deliver, at an accelerating pace, an abundance of previously unimaginable perspectives to help us navigate our future clinical advances. These will be the subjects for future editions.

—*Richard B. Rosen, MD*

Section I
Oculoplastics

Section Editor
Wendy W. Lee, MD, MS

1

EXTERNAL PHOTOGRAPHY

Alexandra E. Levitt, MD, MPH
Apostolos Anagnostopoulos, MD
Wendy W. Lee, MD, MS

External color photography is an important component of any preoperative oculoplastics evaluation, both to document functional impairment as well as to provide a baseline for the patient and surgeon to refer to postoperatively for comparison. External color photographs are typically required by insurance carriers as part of the preoperative evaluation of dermatochalasis, ptosis, or brow ptosis. These photographs are also useful to document eyelid abnormalities such as lower lid ectropion, entropion, or trichiasis, as well as globe positional abnormalities such as proptosis or enophthalmos. They are also essential for telemedicine applications, such as seeking input from an offsite specialist or for second opinions. While the advent of digital photography has greatly simplified the process of image acquisition, not all photographs are equivalent, especially when they must provide critical clinical data. This does not mean that an expensive digital single-lens reflex (DSLR) camera is required to obtain high quality photographs (although in the hands of an experienced photographer one may be particularly helpful). Many smartphone cameras are capable of producing excellent photographs if proper attention is paid to lighting and composition (Figure 1-1).

Small details that may be unimportant in recreational photography are very important in clinical situations. Clinical photographs must be well lit, have the appropriate white balance, and display the pathology of interest in focus and at an angle that highlights its aberration from normal anatomy. Some degree of standardization of these elements of composition is also important to allow accurate and useful comparison between a series of photographs taken over time. There are a few general guidelines to keep in mind when composing a clinical image, which will be explored in more detail later.

Gologorsky D, Rosen RB, eds.
Principles of Ocular Imaging (pp 3-9).
© 2021 Taylor & Francis Group.

Figure 1-1. External color photograph documenting a right lower lid nodule. This nodule developed secondary to an atypical mycobacterial infection following a trans-conjunctival lower lid blepharoplasty. This photograph was obtained with a mobile phone camera, but proper lighting and focus ensure a high-quality image that documents the pathology well. Standardizing the angle of the photograph (eg, either frontal or 45-degree oblique view) would help to ensure that future images could be compared accurately.

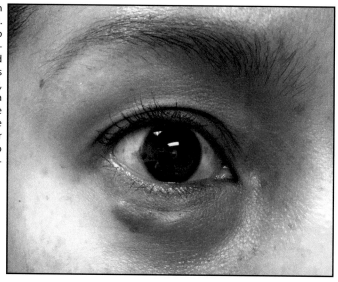

LIGHTING AND COMPOSITION

It is critical for the subject to be appropriately lit. Harsh shadows from overhead lighting may obscure fine details. Similarly, excessive flash illumination along the viewing axis of the camera may overexpose the subject and bleach out more subtle findings. Image clarity is critical and may suffer in dim illumination if the camera is not stabilized or flash is not used to prevent motion artifact.

It is also important to ensure that the camera is accurately focused on the pathology of interest. When using a digital camera with an LCD viewing screen, it may be necessary to zoom in to the detail of interest in order to ensure appropriate focus, relying on the preview function is usually insufficient to determine this. White balance must also be adjusted. Most digital cameras have a set of white balance options to choose from that reduce the blue or yellow cast of different types of indoor lighting. This is particularly important when documenting skin tone, pigmentation, or erythema.

PATIENT POSITIONING

Being mindful of the intended purpose of the photograph is always important. How can the pathology of interest best be demonstrated? If fine details of periocular skin are of interest, documenting before and after a cosmetic laser procedure, a close view with a fine level of focus and detail are important. However, if the goal is to document brow position before and after a coronal brow lift surgery, including a wide-angle view of the face is important for perspective.

The angle of the photograph must also be considered. For example, to document dermatochalasis, both anatomic (straight-on) and oblique views may be useful (Figure 1-2). For these photographs, the patient's head is rotated 45 degrees from the camera axis. Lateral views, with a 90-degree rotation, may also be utilized. In the anatomic and oblique positions, a line drawn from the upper edge of tragus to the inferior-most point of the orbit (the Frankfurt plane) should be horizontal to maintain the appropriate perspective. A frontal view is also useful in documenting lid abnormalities such as entropion and ectropion or full-face pathology (Figures 1-3, 1-4, and 1-5).

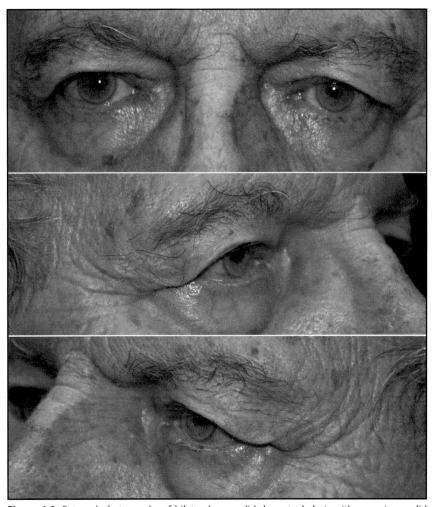

Figure 1-2. External photographs of bilateral upper lid dermatochalasis with excessive eyelid skin touching the eyelashes and obstructing the superior and lateral visual field. Anatomic and oblique views are pictured.

To demonstrate pathology relating to anterior-posterior malposition, such as proptosis or enophthalmos, a basal, or "worm's eye" view is useful (Figure 1-6). As a general guideline, the tip of the nose should be aligned with the brow to standardize the angle of view. However, this may be adjusted based on the clinical scenario. In some cases, such as documenting lagophthalmos, photographs with the eyes both open and closed are useful (Figure 1-7).

REPRODUCIBILITY

Standardization of lighting, positioning, and background are important if a series of images is taken over time (Figure 1-8). Changes in the angle of the photograph, patient positioning (including head tilt), or white balance and lighting make it difficult to accurately assess change over time. Grossly different background colors also distort the perception of foreground color, even under similar lighting conditions, and may be distracting. Background standardization may be achieved

Figure 1-3. External color photographs clearly document bilateral upper lid ptosis and dermatochalasis with fat prolapse in an 81-year-old man with a history of multiple prior lid surgeries. Lower lid retraction with spastic entropion is noted on the left, along with mild conjunctival chemosis and injection. The image is well lit and in focus, and this anatomic view best demonstrates the lid pathology.

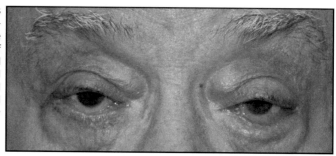

Figure 1-4. This external color photograph documents bilateral involutional ectropion of the lower eyelids. The lid pathology is clearly demonstrated in this photo, although the patient would ideally be looking straight at the camera to better standardize the upper lid position.

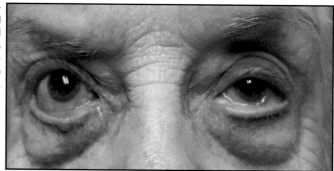

Figure 1-5. External color photograph demonstrating right-sided facial paralysis and droop.

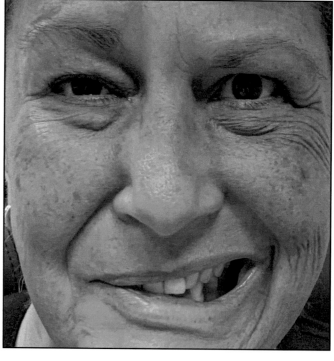

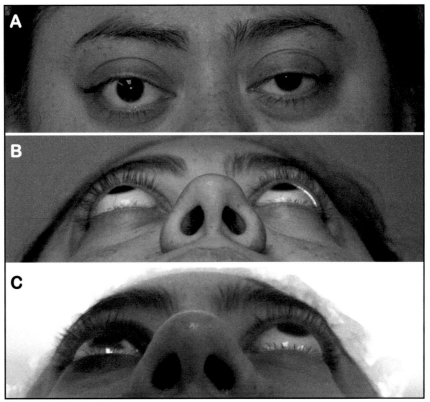

Figure 1-6. External photographs demonstrating bilateral proptosis in a patient with thyroid eye disease. (A) An anatomic view gives an idea of the pathology, (B) but the basal or "worm's eye view" best demonstrates the degree of proptosis, right greater than left. Repeat photographs from a basal view document the improvement after right-sided orbital decompression prior to subsequent decompression of the left orbit. (C) Note the tip of the nose aligned with the brow helps standardize the angle of the photograph and aids in obtaining images that are useful for comparison. Ideally, the image in panel C would be enhanced with removal of the patient's hair-net and the addition of a solid color background similar to that in the prior panels.

by positioning a patient against a solid color wall (black, white, or muted blue are popular choices), or placing a poster board behind the patient's head if seated in an exam chair. In the operating room, extraneous surgical implements, hands of assistants, and free tissue and blood should be removed from the shot if at all possible.

PREOPERATIVE PTOSIS AND DERMATOCHALASIS REPAIR

External color photography is specifically required by Medicare to document preexisting dermatochalasis and ptosis. There are a few particular pieces of information that are useful to capture in this scenario, which are described below.

With respect to the preoperative evaluation of ptosis, the margin-reflex distance 1 (MRD1) measurement is the distance from the upper eyelid margin to the center of the cornea. Typically, this must be less than 2 mm to constitute functional ptosis. A properly aligned camera flash eliciting a centered corneal light reflex is thus a very useful element of these photographs (Figure 1-9). With regards to dermatochalasis, the skin of the eyelids is typically required to be resting on the

Figure 1-7. External color photographs documenting cicatricial lagophthalmos of the right eye. Anatomic views, with eyelids both opened and closed, best demonstrates this pathology.

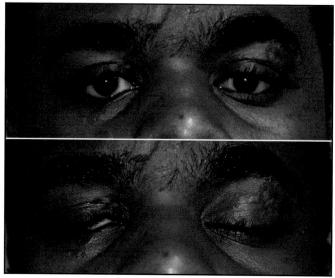

Figure 1-8. (A) External color photographs demonstrating post-traumatic facial scarring with resultant cicatricial ectropion and lagophthalmos. (B) Significant improvements in lid position, skin color, and texture are seen following several sessions of ablative fractional laser resurfacing.

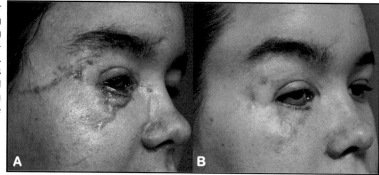

upper eyelashes, or with significant edema, to constitute functionally significant dermatochalasis. If dermatochalasis and ptosis are concurrent, often additional photographs with the excess skin taped up to better assess the position of the lid margin are required (Figure 1-10).

As discussed above, it is important for the patient to be photographed in a sufficiently and evenly lit environment, and for him or her to be positioned perpendicular to the plane of the camera without head tilt. Similarly, it is important for the muscles of the forehead to be relaxed in order to assess the true position of the upper lid. Photographs should not be taken after the application of phenylephrine eye drops (for pharmacologic dilation or otherwise), as this may temporarily raise the position of the upper lid by stimulating the contraction of Müller's muscle.

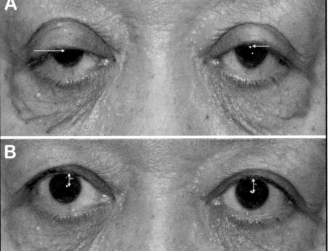

Figure 1-9. External photographs documenting bilateral upper lid ptosis with (A) an MRD1 of 0 mm in the right eye and 0.5 mm in the left eye and (B) an MRD1 of 4 mm in both eyes 5 minutes after instilling phenylephrine 2.5% drops. Phenylephrine drops simulate the effect of ptosis repair. MRD1 indicated with the yellow arrow.

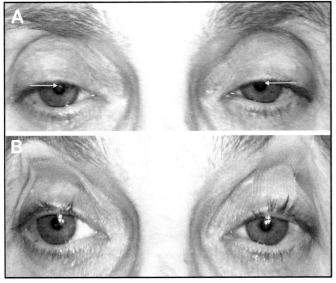

Figure 1-10. (A) External photograph documenting bilateral upper lid ptosis without tape. The MRD1 (yellow arrow), the distance from the upper lid to the corneal light reflex, is 0 mm (no light reflex is visible). (B) With tape to simulate the position of the eyelid after surgery, there is an improvement in MRD1 of 2 mm in both eyes.

2

PTOSIS VISUAL FIELDS

Alexandra E. Levitt, MD, MPH
Apostolos Anagnostopoulos, MD
Ann Q. Tran, MD
Wendy W. Lee, MD, MS

Preoperative evaluation for blepharoplasty, ptosis, or brow ptosis repair typically involves a clinic visit where visual fields, external color photography, and clinical measurements are obtained, as described in the previous chapter. These imaging modalities are important to objectively demonstrate impairment and for the justification of a functional (rather than cosmetic) eyelid or brow surgery, which is important if seeking insurance coverage. In general, a patient must report subjective complaints in association with ptosis or dermatochalasis, such as a restricted visual field, difficulty with performing activities of daily living such as reading or driving, or intractable ocular irritation. The objective testing and imaging must corroborate these claims.

While an in-depth review of visual fields will feature in the Glaucoma section (Chapter 20), this discussion will focus on its use in oculoplastics in the evaluation of ptosis. Visual field testing is undertaken to demonstrate that a significant visual field defect exists and that this defect may be corrected with surgical repair. Each eye is tested first with the eyelid and eyelid skin in their natural position to document the visual field before intervention. Then, tape is applied to mechanically lift the redundant eyelid skin (if considered a candidate for blepharoplasty) or the eyelid margin itself (if considered a candidate for concurrent ptosis repair) to a normal anatomic position in order to estimate the improvement in the visual field after correction. The brows may be manually lifted if brow ptosis is a concern. To qualify for insurance coverage as a functional surgery, the visual field must typically improve by a minimum of 12 degrees or 30%, depending on the type of visual field performed.

Traditional Humphrey visual field testing used commonly in glaucoma or neuro-ophthalmic indications may be used in this setting, although it may not be sufficiently sensitive to detect all clinically significant superior visual field defects. The modified Leicester visual field test was specifically designed to assess ptosis and dermatochalasis, and is commonly used in this application.

Gologorsky D, Rosen RB, eds.
Principles of Ocular Imaging (pp 11-16).
© 2021 Taylor & Francis Group.

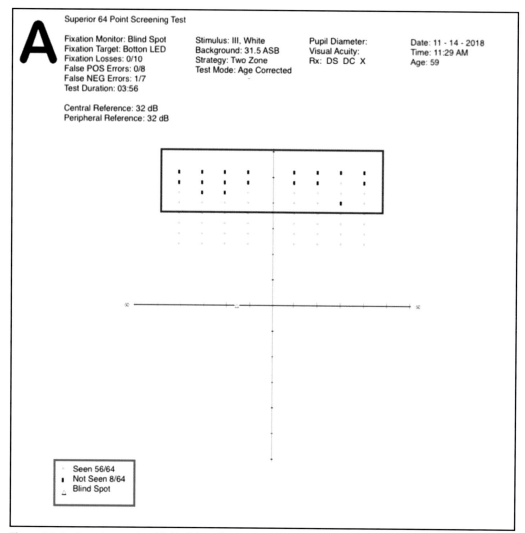

Figure 2-1. Static perimetry visual field of the right eye (A) without tape (56/64 points seen) and (B) with tape (46/56 points seen) for a patient with upper lid dermatochalasis. Although the testing with tape shows an improvement of 10 points in the superior visual field, it does not qualify as functional dermatochalasis based on Medicare standards of >30% degrees of improvement. Points not seen are those in black within the red box in each part of the figure. (*continued*)

This test was first described as assessing 35 points in the superior 48 degrees of the visual field, with 14 inferior points included as reference. Modified versions of this test add additional points to more fully characterize the superior visual field (Figures 2-1 and 2-2). This automated test has the benefit of being relatively fast, easy to perform, and operator independent. A minimum of a 30% improvement in the points seen in the superior visual field is necessary to qualify as functional for the majority of insurance providers.

Goldmann visual fields and other types of dynamic perimetry such as tangent screen testing are also commonly used to assess the superior visual field before eyelid surgery (Figure 2-3). This method provides a better assessment of the far periphery at the expense of taking more time and

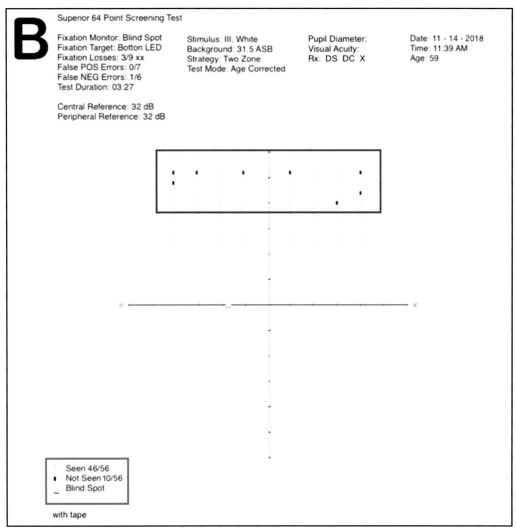

Figure 2-1 (continued). Static perimetry visual field of the right eye (A) without tape (56/64 points seen) and (B) with tape (46/56 points seen) for a patient with upper lid dermatochalasis. Although the testing with tape shows an improvement of 10 points in the superior visual field, it does not qualify as functional dermatochalasis based on Medicare standards of >30% degrees of improvement. Points not seen are those in black within the red box in each part of the figure.

requiring a skilled operator to administer. To perform a Goldmann visual field, the patient fixates on a central target in the center of a white hemisphere. The examiner moves a lighted target in from the periphery toward the center point, and the patient indicates when the target is in view by pressing a buzzer. This process is repeated to map out the limits of a patient's visual field. A 12% improvement in the degrees of superior visual field is typically required to constitute a functional impairment. In a patient with complaints of a visual field defect and symptomatic ptosis or dermatochalasis who fails to qualify based on a conventional or Leicester visual field, the Goldmann or other types of dynamic perimetry, if available, may better capture the patient's complaints.

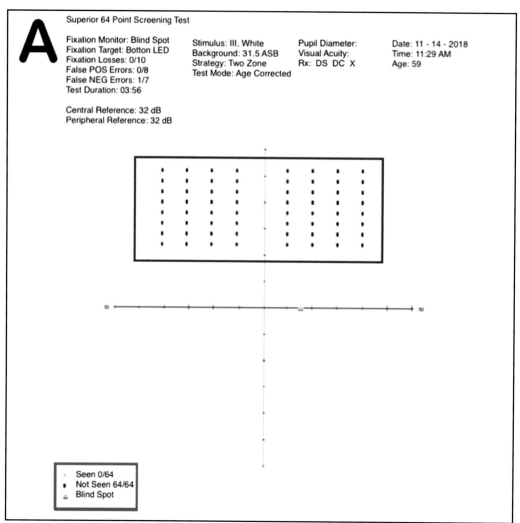

Figure 2-2. Static perimetry visual field of the right eye (A) without tape (0/64 points seen) for a patient with upper lid ptosis, >30% degrees of improvement, qualifying for functional upper lid ptosis surgery. Points not seen are those in black within the red box in each part of the figure. (*continued*)

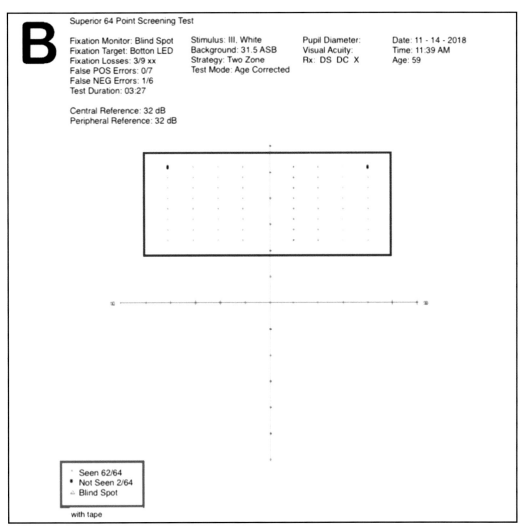

Figure 2-2 (continued). Static perimetry visual field of the right eye (B) with tape (62/64 points seen) for a patient with upper lid ptosis, > 30% degrees of improvement, qualifying for functional upper lid ptosis surgery. Points not seen are those in black within the red box in each part of the figure.

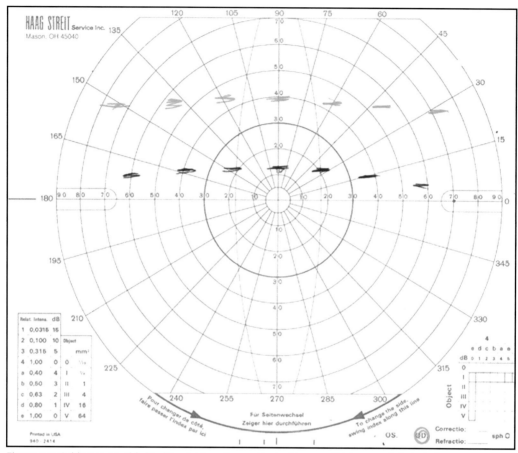

Figure 2-3. Goldmann visual field of the right eye for a patient with upper lid dermatochalasis. It shows an improvement of 26 degrees (from 13 at the purple line to 39 degrees the green line) which is > 12 degrees, or 30%, and qualifies as functional upper lid dermatochalasis.

3

SLIT LAMP PHOTOGRAPHY

Ashwinee Ragam, MD

A slit lamp is a powerful microscope that provides eye doctors with a magnified, stereoscopic view of the anterior segment and ocular adnexa. This device couples a binocular viewing system with a pivoting illumination source, whose beam height, width, color, and intensity can be adjusted by the operator. Broad, on-axis illumination offers a large, even field of view of the anterior segment with bright colors, but flattened images. Thin, off-axis illumination improves the apparent depth of focus, providing an optical cross-section of the cornea, along with a detailed view of intraocular structures. Most slit lamps offer a range of magnification from 6x to 40x.

There are specific techniques of adjusting a slit lamp to optimize imaging of select anatomic features. Diffuse illumination employs a wide light beam of medium intensity onto the eye at 45 degrees or less from the microscope, primarily to provide an overall image of the front of the eye. Optical sectioning is accomplished using a narrow, high-intensity light beam positioned at a 45- to 60-degree angle; it reveals elevations of the conjunctiva and sclera, and shows the cornea, the anterior chamber, and lens in cross-section. Sclerotic scatter utilizes a wide, bright beam focused onto the limbal sclera; light travels laterally through the cornea by means of total internal reflection to indirectly illuminate otherwise seemingly transparent opacities. Retroillumination is accomplished by shining an axial beam (parallel to the microscope) through a dilated pupil to highlight corneal and lenticular opacities against the retinal red reflex. Transillumination similarly reflects an axial light beam through an undilated pupil and off of the retina to illuminate iris defects.

Slit lamp microscopes are core instrumentation in the eye examination lane. As electronic recordkeeping becomes increasingly the standard of care, the demand for documentational imaging of eye exam findings will become more common. Cameras can be mounted on slit lamps (Figure 3-1) so that the examiner can capture their view through the microscope by simply pressing a button or a foot pedal. Light entering the microscope can be partially diverted to the

Gologorsky D, Rosen RB, eds.
Principles of Ocular Imaging (pp 17-26).
© 2021 Taylor & Francis Group.

Figure 3-1. A Hitachi camera mounted to a slit lamp microscope. Photographs are captured by a foot pedal.

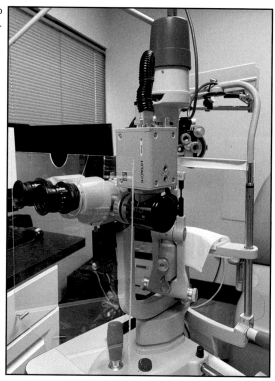

camera using a beam splitter or completely reflected into the camera using a movable mirror. A fill-in flash accessory can help to even out the lighting of the image by filling in shadows in the background of the illuminated beam. Without this illumination adjustment, the slit beam would appear to be floating in a dark void. Slit lamp photography is highly beneficial in documenting pathology and monitoring disease progression and/or response to treatment by means of serial imaging. Furthermore, photographs can aid in sharing the examination experience with other providers as well as informing patients about their ocular condition. More recently, smartphones are being employed for quick and immediately accessible slit lamp photography by aligning the phone cameras with the microscope oculars.

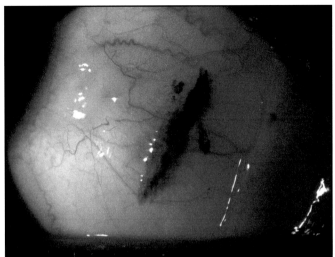

Figure 3-2. Slit lamp photograph using diffuse illumination to show a nasal bulbar conjunctival pigmented lesion.

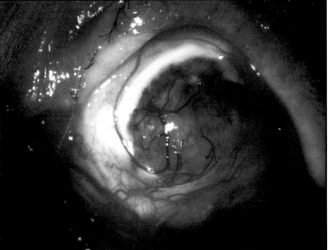

Figure 3-3. Slit lamp photograph using optical sectioning to show an active superotemporal scleral melt with uveal protrusion in the right eye of a patient with rheumatoid arthritis.

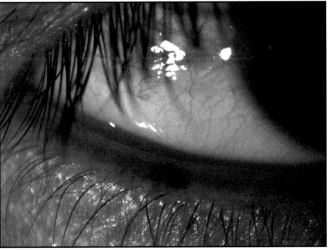

Figure 3-4. Slit lamp photograph using diffuse illumination to show a pigmented lower eyelid lesion.

Figure 3-5. Slit lamp photograph using diffuse illumination to show epithelial ingrowth after LASIK.

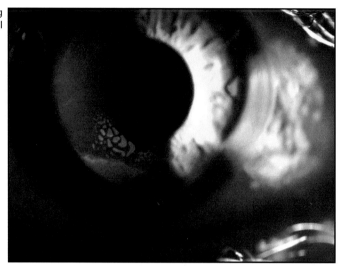

Figure 3-6. Slit lamp photograph using diffuse cobalt blue light to illuminate a corneal epithelial dendrite, which stains with fluorescein dye.

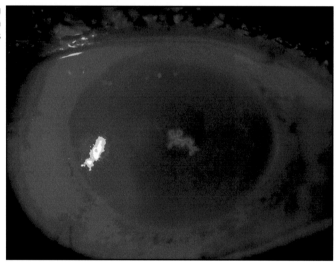

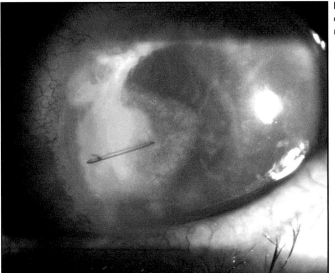

Figure 3-7. Slit lamp photograph using diffuse illumination to show a suture-related corneal ulcer.

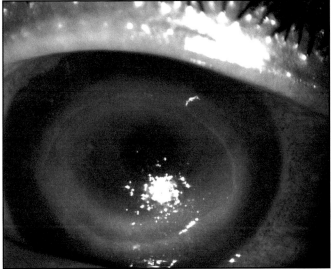

Figure 3-8. Slit lamp photograph using diffuse illumination to show a suspected case of *Acanthamoeba* keratitis.

Figure 3-9. Slit lamp photograph using diffuse illumination to show a Fuchs' adenoma (benign ciliary body tumor).

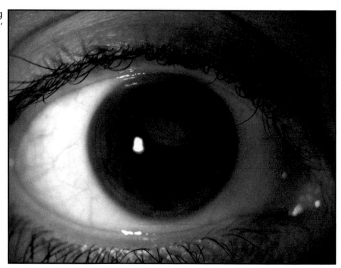

Figure 3-10. Slit lamp photograph using diffuse illumination to show a pigmented iris lesion.

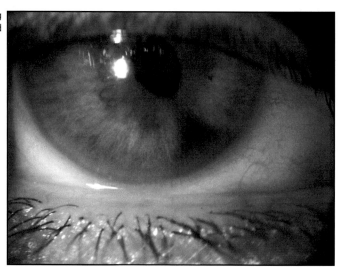

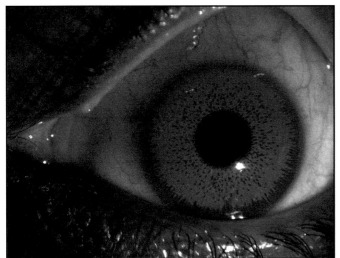

Figure 3-11. Slit lamp photograph using diffuse illumination to show an artificial iris implant.

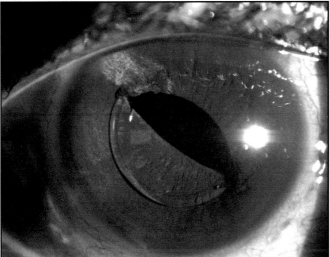

Figure 3-12. Slit lamp photograph using diffuse illumination to show an intraocular lens with the inferior half of the optic being captured over the iris.

Figure 3-13. Slit lamp photograph of a posterior polar cataract, demonstrated by retroillumination.

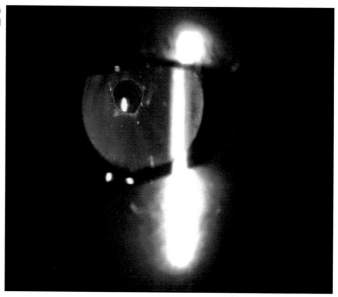

Figure 3-14. Slit lamp photograph using optical sectioning showing crystalline stromal dystrophy.

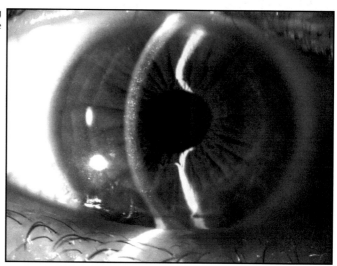

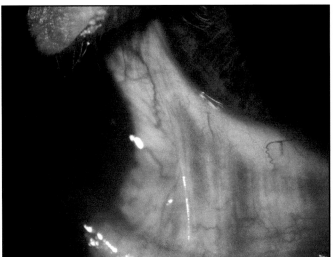

Figure 3-15. Slit lamp photograph using diffuse illumination to show symblepharon in the inferior fornix.

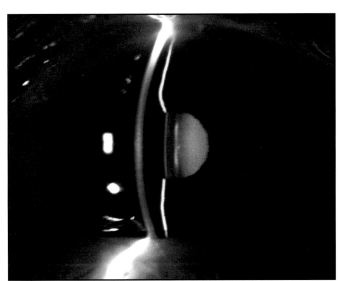

Figure 3-16. Slit lamp photograph using optical sectioning to show a dense nuclear cataract. The thin light beam illuminates a cross-section of the crystalline lens, delineating its layers (from anterior to posterior): capsule, cortex, and nucleus.

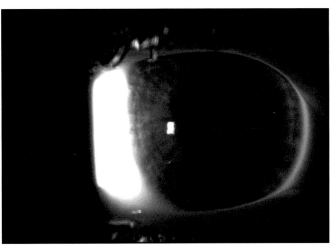

Figure 3-17. Slit lamp photograph showing the sclerotic scatter examination technique.

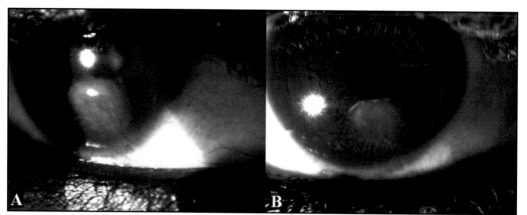

Figure 3-18. Slit lamp photographs of an inflammatory corneal nodule (A) before and (B) after treatment with topical corticosteroids. The regression of blood vessels from the nodule can be easily appreciated using side-by-side images.

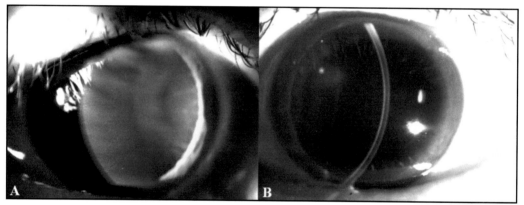

Figure 3-19. Slit lamp photographs of a patient with diffuse corneal haze. (A) The pathology was localized to the pre-Descemet's level by the use of a thin beam (B) to examine the corneal cross-section.

4

ORBITAL ULTRASONOGRAPHY

Ying Chen, MD
Andrew J. Rong, MD
Amy Huang, BS
John Hinkle, MD
Nimesh Patel, MD
Wendy W. Lee, MD, MS

Ultrasound is an important imaging modality and diagnostic tool for ocular and orbital pathology. Ocular ultrasound uses high-frequency sound waves; these sound waves penetrate tissue and then are reflected, leading to the vibration of a piezoelectric crystal in the transducer. These vibrations generate electrical signals that are translated into images and other information. Lower frequency sound waves have lower resolution but greater tissue penetration, allowing for evaluation of deep structures. Higher frequency sound waves have less tissue penetration but higher resolution, making them ideal for the evaluation of superficial structures. Factors that affect returning sound waves or echoes include differences between tissue mediums (interface between tissue types), density, and the angle at which a transducer is held.

Several different ultrasound modes exist and include A-, B-, M-, and Doppler-modes. The A-mode, or *amplitude mode*, generates a one-dimensional graphical representation of reflected sound waves in the form of amplitudes or "spikes," which correspond to different tissue interfaces (Figure 4-1). The more dissimilar two tissue mediums are, the larger the spike. On the contrary, the more similar two tissue mediums are, the smaller the spike. Denser mediums also absorb more energy and decrease spike height. Characteristics such as reflectivity (absolute spike height), internal structure (spike height regularity), and sound attenuation (spike height angle of decline) can provide information about tissue makeup and aid in the diagnosis of pathology. The B-mode, or *brightness mode*, generates a two-dimensional image, where reflected sound waves are converted into points of varying brightness that correspond to echo amplitude (Figure 4-2). Higher amplitude echoes will appear brighter or hyperechoic, while lower amplitude echoes will appear dimmer or hypoechoic. The M-mode, or *motion mode*, generates a two-dimensional image with recorded motions. The Doppler mode is used to measure blood flow and evaluate vascular

Gologorsky D, Rosen RB, eds.
Principles of Ocular Imaging (pp 27-33).
© 2021 Taylor & Francis Group.

Figure 4-1. A-scan. Peaks represent different interfaces, as identified in the image.

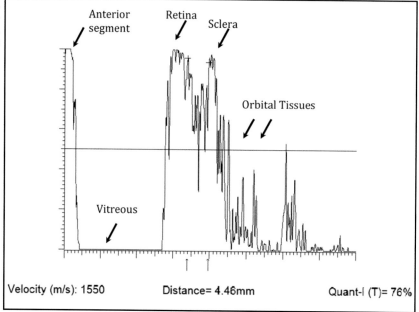

lesions. The Doppler effect describes the phenomenon of a perceived frequency change when an observer is moving relative to the wave source. The Doppler mode can measure blood velocity and flow via Doppler frequency shifts of reflected sound waves from moving red blood cells. Continuous wave, pulsed wave, and color flow are subtypes of Doppler ultrasound. The Duplex mode combines the B-mode and Doppler mode to visualize and measure blood flow. Ultrasound biomicroscopy (UBM) is a high-frequency ophthalmic ultrasound that uses 50 MHz sound waves and is particularly helpful in examining the anterior segment given the high-resolution images it provides (Figure 4-3). However, it is limited to the examination of anterior segment structures.

Ultrasound is performed by systematically examining the eye in two essential planes, transverse (probe parallel to the limbus) and longitudinal (probe perpendicular to the limbus). Prior to the exam, an anesthetic drop is placed into the eye, and ophthalmic tear gel is used as a coupling medium for the ultrasound probe. The ultrasound probe is then placed directly on the globe with the probe marker oriented in the desired direction (Figure 4-4). In ophthalmology, ultrasound is typically used for the following purposes:

- Evaluation of intraocular pathology when opaque media obstructs the fundus and posterior pole (eg, retinal detachments [see Figure 4-2], intraocular foreign bodies, or optic nerve disorders [Figure 4-5])

- Evaluation of extraocular anatomy and pathology (eg, extraocular muscles or retrobulbar space)

- Preoperative axial length measurement for intraocular lens power calculations and cataract surgery (Figure 4-6)

Ultrasound is useful because it is low cost, safe, and provides information in real time. However, it has a significant amount of interoperator variability.

Orbital ultrasound can rapidly aid in the diagnosis of different diseases, such as orbital masses, vascular lesions, and extraocular diseases. Ultrasound can evaluate orbital masses including orbital lymphoma and rhabdomyosarcoma. Lymphomas can present as irregularly shaped, hypoechoic masses with low internal reflectivity and weak sound attenuation on A- and B-scan (Figure 4-7). Rhabdomyosarcoma can present as irregularly shaped, hypoechoic masses with irregular inter-

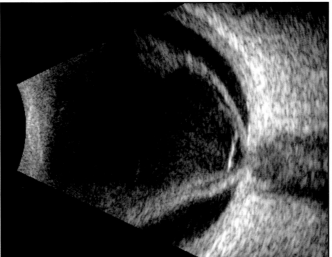

Figure 4-2. B-scan of a retinal detachment.

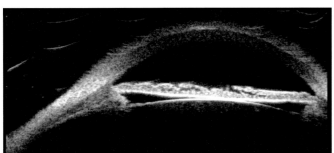

Figure 4-3. UBM of the anterior segment anatomy.

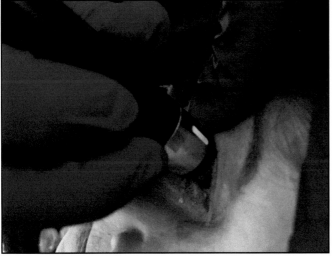

Figure 4-4. Performing an ultrasound of the globe and orbit. The probe is over the eye with coupling agent.

nal reflectivity on A- and B-scan (Figure 4-8). Ultrasound can even detect rare diseases such as Rosai-Dorfman disease, characterized by nonmalignant proliferation of histiocytes within lymph node sinuses and other extranodal sites, such as the orbit (Figure 4-9). Orbital ultrasound, especially Doppler ultrasound, can also be useful in evaluating vascular lesions. Capillary heman-

Figure 4-5. B-scan evaluation of the optic nerve on ultrasound.

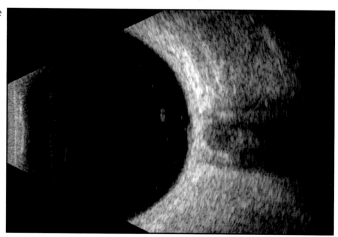

Figure 4-6. Preoperative axial length measurement for intraocular lens power calculations and cataract surgery.

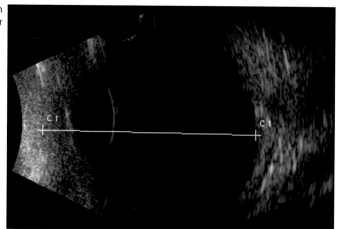

Figure 4-7. B-scan of orbital lymphoma demonstrating an irregularly shaped, hypoechoic mass with low internal reflectivity and weak sound attenuation.

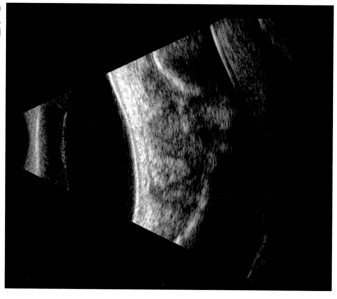

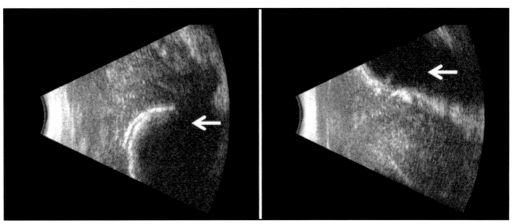

Figure 4-8. B-scans of an orbital rhabdomyosarcoma showing a nodular, hypoechoic mass with irregular internal reflectivity.

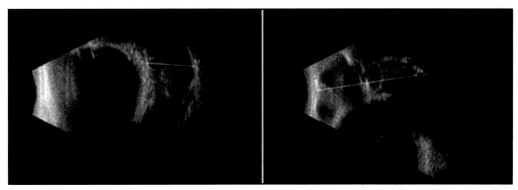

Figure 4-9. B-scan of Rosai-Dorfman disease involving the orbit. Irregularly shaped, well-defined, mildly compressible, moderately vascular masses with septae and low reflectivity shown in two different views.

giomas, the most common orbital vascular tumor in infants, can present as irregularly shaped, hyperechoic, compressible, vascularized masses with high reflectivity and sound attenuation on A- and B-scan (Figure 4-10). Cavernous malformations, the most common orbital lesions in adults, can present as hyperechoic masses with high internal reflectivity due to their pseudocapsules on A- and B-scan. Other vascular lesions include orbital varices, which appear distensible during the Valsalva maneuver and may show blood flow reversal on Doppler ultrasound, and lymphangiomas, which can present as multiple fluid-filled, non-vascularized cysts (Figure 4-11).

Ultrasound can also detect extraocular manifestations of disease such as extraocular muscle enlargement, which is most commonly caused by thyroid orbitopathy, orbital myositis, and orbital venous congestion. In thyroid eye disease (TED), orbital muscle bellies can be enlarged, but muscle insertions are typically spared (Figure 4-12). On ultrasound, the muscles typically have high reflectivity especially when they have become fibrotic in late stages of disease (Figure 4-13). Orbital myositis can be differentiated from TED by muscle insertion involvement and reduced muscle belly reflectivity. Depending on the extent of inflammation, a "T-sign," or fluid in Tenon's space, can be seen when posterior scleritis is present (Figure 4-14). Finally, in congestive orbital disorders such as carotid-cavernous fistulas, there is vascular engorgement of the extraocular muscles but no change in muscle echogenicity. Other findings such as an enlarged superior ophthalmic vein or abnormal blood flow on Doppler ultrasound may be detected. In these ways, disease progression and treatment response may be monitored using these ultrasound findings.

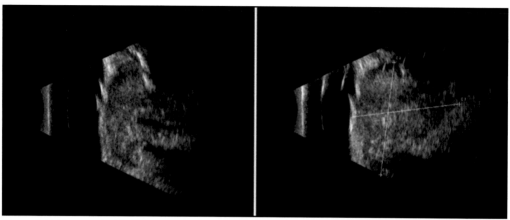

Figure 4-10. B-scans of orbital hemangioma demonstrating an irregularly shaped, hyperechoic, compressible, vascularized mass with high reflectivity and sound attenuation shown in two different views.

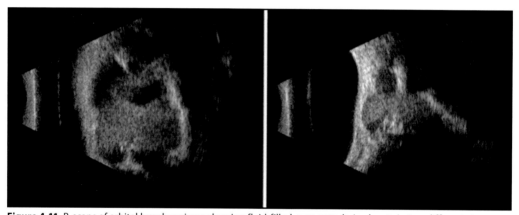

Figure 4-11. B-scans of orbital lymphangioma showing fluid-filled, non-vascularized cysts in two different views.

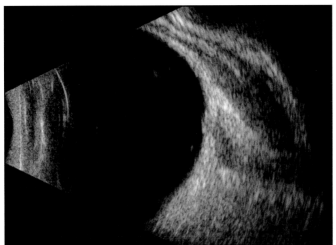

Figure 4-12. B-scan of muscle belly enlargement without muscle insertion involvement in TED.

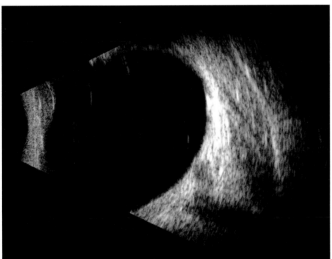

Figure 4-13. B-scan of muscle belly enlargement with high reflectivity in late stage TED.

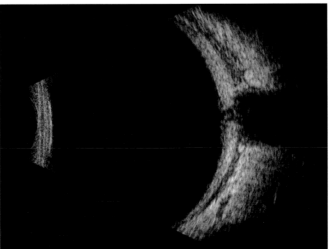

Figure 4-14. B-scan of T-sign (fluid in Tenon's space) in posterior scleritis.

Section II
Cornea and Refractive

Section Editors
Ashwinee Ragam, MD
Oriel Spierer, MD

5

Corneal Topography

Ashwinee Ragam, MD

Corneal topography is an imaging technique utilized for assessing the shape, curvature, and thickness of the cornea. Clinical uses of corneal topography include characterizing and quantifying keratometric astigmatism (both of the native cornea and post-keratoplasty), screening for and monitoring progressive corneal ectasia, and evaluating surgical candidates for premium intraocular lenses and laser vision correction. There are three methods of obtaining corneal topography: Placido disc-based imaging (eg, Atlas [Carl Zeiss Meditec, Inc], OPD-Scan [Nidek, Inc]), scanning slit imaging (eg, Orbscan [Bausch & Lomb]), and Scheimpflug imaging (eg, Pentacam [Oculus, Inc], Galilei [Ziemer Ophthalmic Systems]).

PLACIDO DISC-BASED IMAGING

First developed in the 19th century, the Placido disc technique involves projecting a series of concentric rings onto the anterior corneal surface and then measuring the reflection of these rings, called *mires*. A perfect cornea should demonstrate concentric, spherical mires equally spaced over the surface. Mires that appear more closely together indicate areas of corneal steepening while areas of more widely spaced mires represent a flatter cornea. Ovoid mires may suggest regular astigmatism, while wavy or distorted mires can indicate ocular surface disease or irregular astigmatism. This imaging technique is highly dependent on the integrity of the tear film from which the light is actually being reflected.

Placido disc technology has evolved from purely qualitative keratoscopy to quantitative topography. Corneal slope values can be directly measured at thousands of points along the mires and converted by an algorithm to curvature values in millimeters. Curvature values may then

Gologorsky D, Rosen RB, eds.
Principles of Ocular Imaging (pp 37-44).
© 2021 Taylor & Francis Group.

be converted to refractive power values in diopters (D) using a simple formula incorporating the refractive index of the anterior cornea (1.3375). Placido disc technology cannot assess the posterior corneal surface.

SCANNING SLIT IMAGING

These topographers perform two vertical scans by projecting light through optical slits at fixed angles to the cornea. Light reflected back is captured by a camera and analyzed by a reference slit beam to generate information on both the anterior and posterior corneal curvatures. Imaging the posterior corneal curvature independently is critical for detecting early ectasia patterns as well as for analyzing post-refractive eyes in which the anterior corneal surfaces have been ablated. Scanning slit topographers can additionally generate information on corneal thickness and elevation.

SCHEIMPFLUG IMAGING

In this technique, a camera perpendicular to a slit beam creates optical sections between the cornea and the lens. The camera can be rotated to generate a three-dimensional model of the anterior segment from which all topographic information is derived. Similar to scanning slit topography, Scheimpflug cameras can image the posterior cornea and measure corneal elevation. However, Scheimpflug technology has been shown to have higher repeatability of corneal measurements than scanning slit technology.

The Pentacam uses one rotating Scheimpflug camera and one static camera, the latter of which is centered over the pupil and controls patient fixation. The Galilei integrates dual rotating Scheimpflug cameras with Placido disc technology.

INTERPRETATION OF CORNEAL TOPOGRAPHY

Most topography used today will report the central (3 to 5 mm) steepest and flattest corneal points. These points can be measured from the anterior and posterior corneal surfaces separately. The degree of corneal astigmatism is calculated as the difference between the central flattest and steepest points. Central corneal points greater than 47 D and astigmatism greater than 6 D are concerning for ectasia.

Sometimes reported is the Q-value, which represents the overall asphericity of the cornea. A Q-value of zero indicates a perfectly spherical shape. Negative Q-values denote the normal prolate nature of the human cornea, whose center is steep with flattening toward the periphery. The average Q-value for human corneas is -0.26. Eyes that have undergone myopic ablation often become oblate in shape (flat at the apex with steepening towards the periphery) and have a positive Q-value.

Different maps can be generated of the imaged cornea. Color scales are placed next to the maps to guide interpretation. Each map provides unique data and additional clues to understanding the overall corneal topography:

- The *axial curvature map*, also known as the *sagittal curvature map*, displays dioptric values of the anterior corneal surface. Steeper areas (higher dioptric values) are displayed as warmer colors while flatter areas (lower dioptric values) are displayed as cooler colors. Axial maps most accurately represent the central curvature but assume peripheral points to fit within a "smooth" map of the corneal surface. Axial maps are best used to characterize corneal astigmatism. Regular astigmatism shows a "bow tie" or "figure-of-eight pattern" of steepening along a single meridian, with symmetric halves across the corneal center. With-the-rule regular astigmatism is steep within 30 degrees of the vertical meridian (90 degrees), while against-the-rule astigmatism is steep within 30 degrees of the horizontal meridian (180 degrees). Oblique regular astigmatism is steep somewhere between 30 and 60 degrees or 120 and 150 degrees.

- The *tangential curvature map*, also known as *instantaneous map*, also displays dioptric values of the anterior corneal surface, but is based on the radius of curvature at individual points measured at 90-degree tangents. As such, it gives a truer depiction of the peripheral cornea than would an axial map. Because tangential maps are sensitive to small changes in curvature, they may be considered too detailed, if not "noisy," and therefore less useful in quick screenings for corneal astigmatism and ectasia.

- The *corneal thickness map* displays pachymetry values in micrometers, with warmer colors representing thinner areas and cooler colors representing thicker areas.

- The *elevation maps*, also known as *floats*, define the height of the cornea in micrometers by generating a computerized best-fit sphere that matches the average measured corneal curvature in a central inclusion zone (usually 7 to 8 mm). Elevation maps are produced for the anterior and posterior corneal surfaces separately. Warmer colors represent areas of the true cornea that are elevated above the best-fit sphere while cooler colors represent areas that are depressed below the best-fit sphere. These maps can be helpful in identifying early ectasia as well as predicting contact lens fit.

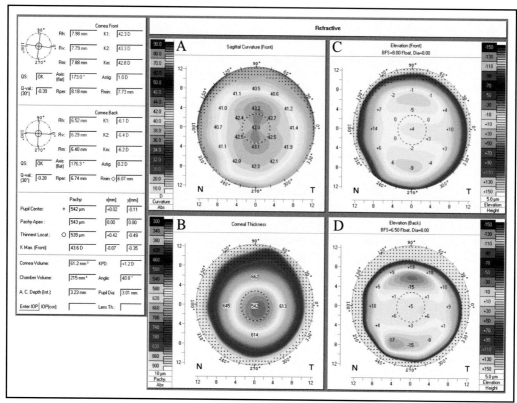

Figure 5-1. Pentacam refractive panel of a normal right eye. (A) Axial map of the anterior cornea demonstrates regular (symmetric "bow tie") with-the-rule astigmatism, steep along approximately the 90-degree meridian. (B) Pachymetry map. (C) Anterior elevation ("float") map. (D) Posterior elevation ("float") map.

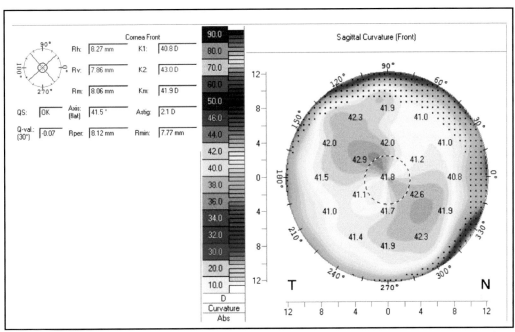

Figure 5-2. Pentacam axial map of a right eye with regular (symmetric "bow tie") oblique astigmatism, steep along approximately the 130-degree meridian. The flat meridian is identified in the key (41.5 degrees), and in regular astigmatism the steep meridian should be 90 degrees away.

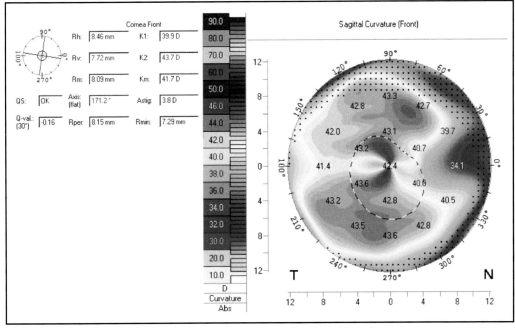

Figure 5-3. Pentacam axial map of a right eye with pterygium-induced nasal flattening.

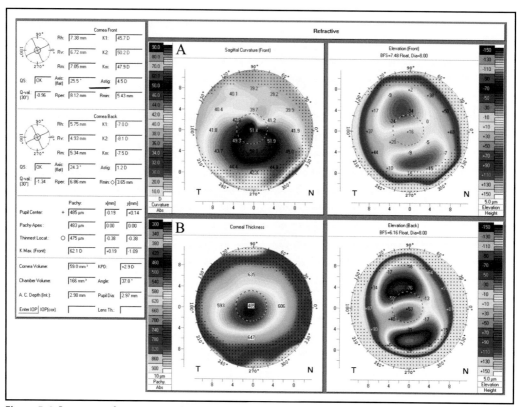

Figure 5-4. Pentacam refractive panel of a right eye keratoconus. (A) Axial map of the anterior cornea demonstrates 4.5 D of irregular astigmatism with the inferior half of the "bow tie" steeper than the superior half. The steepest central point is 50.2 D. (B) Pachymetry map demonstrates that the thinnest central point is 475 μm.

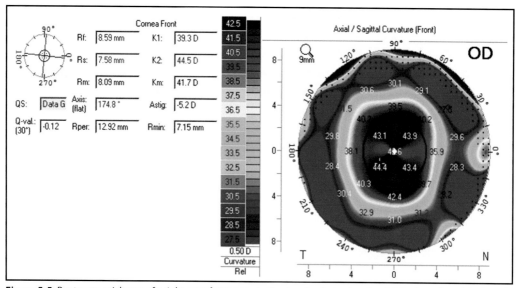

Figure 5-5. Pentacam axial map of a right eye after a penetrating keratoplasty showing 5.2 D of regular, with-the-rule astigmatism (steep along approximately the 85-degree meridian). A pair of tight sutures were subsequently removed from the 6 and 12 o'clock positions.

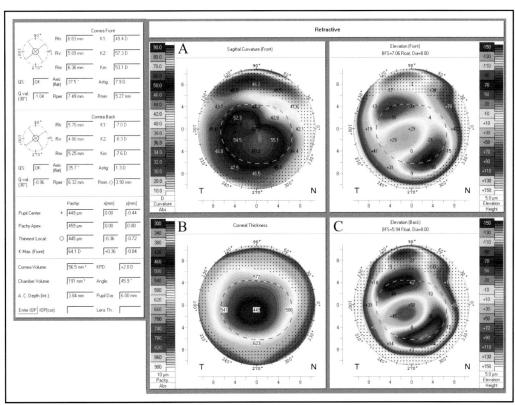

Figure 5-6. Pentacam refractive panel of a right eye keratoconus. (A) Axial map of the anterior cornea demonstrates 7.9 D of irregular astigmatism with the inferior half of the "bow tie" steeper than the superior half. The steepest central point is 60.2 D. (B) Pachymetry map shows that the thinnest central point is 445 μm. (C) Posterior "float" map shows paracentral bulges, greatest inferiorly, above the best-fit sphere, which is consistent with keratoconus.

Figure 5-7. Pentacam axial map of a right eye with irregular ocular surface and tear film abnormalities.

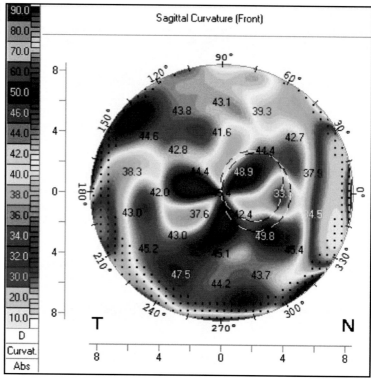

6

CONFOCAL MICROSCOPY

Ashwinee Ragam, MD

Confocal microscopy allows for non-invasive, *in vivo* visualization of all layers of the cornea. The technique involves directly illuminating and observing a source at the same focal point and utilizing pinholes to block excess out-of-focus light, which degrades image quality. What results is an image with high resolution and magnification but a very limited field of view; therefore, several points must be synchronously captured to produce a clinically useful image. The current primary clinical application of confocal microscopy is in imaging the corneal endothelium; some suggest it may gradually replace specular microscopy for the purpose of obtaining an endothelial cell count.

The corneal endothelium is a monolayer of hexagonal cells which image as homogeneously bright cytoplasm with clearly defined dark cell borders. Endothelial cells serve a critical role in maintaining corneal clarity by acting as a physical barrier to aqueous humor and functioning as desiccating metabolic pumps. These cells do not regenerate, so tracking their density and viability is important in assessing the health of native and transplanted corneal tissue. As endothelial cells die, which happens naturally with age or at an accelerated rate in the setting of trauma or disease, the remaining cells expand to fill the void and subsequently lose their hexagonal shape. Furthermore, endothelial cell loss and stress leads to the formation of guttae, which are collagenous excrescences of the endothelial basement membrane, Descemet's membrane.

Once a frame of endothelial cells of a known area is captured by the confocal microscope, the examiner can produce data on total cell density by manually counting the cells in the frame and extrapolating the volume/millimeter squared, or by using automated software analysis of cell borders and morphologies. The average endothelial cell count in a 65-year-old healthy eye is around 2500 cells/mm^2. Corneas with fewer than 1000 cells/mm^2 are at greater risk for endothelial decompensation following intraocular surgery. Polymegathism describes increased variation in endothelial cell size, which occurs during cell loss as described previously, but can also be seen

Gologorsky D, Rosen RB, eds.
Principles of Ocular Imaging (pp 45-49).
© 2021 Taylor & Francis Group.

in patients with long-term contact lens wear or diabetes. Pleomorphism describes increased variability in endothelial cell shape; corneas with fewer than 50% hexagonal cells are at a greater risk for decompensation following intraocular surgery.

Confocal microscopy can also be used to assess more anterior corneal pathology including microbial keratitis and stromal depositions and dystrophies. Most confocal microscopes require a coupling media by means of gel immersion to image the entire corneal infrastructure from the epithelium to the endothelium. Non-contact modes exist, but they produce lower magnification images and their utility is limited to viewing the corneal endothelium.

Figure 6-1. Confocal microscopy of a healthy endothelial cell layer. The cells are mostly uniform in size and shape (hexagonal). The cell density was counted as 2405 cells/mm^2.

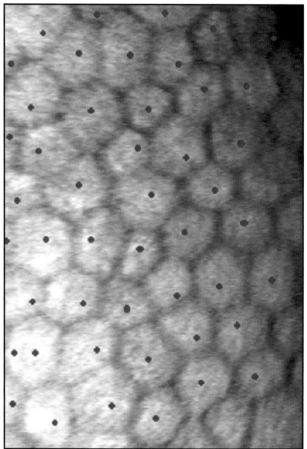

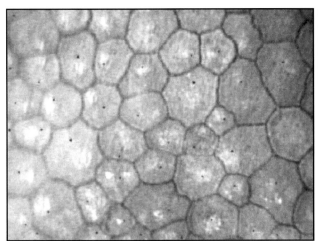

Figure 6-2. Confocal microscopy of early endothelial decompensation. Note that some endothelial cells are larger than others (polymegathism) and many cells do not have a normal hexagonal, six-sided shape (pleomorphism).

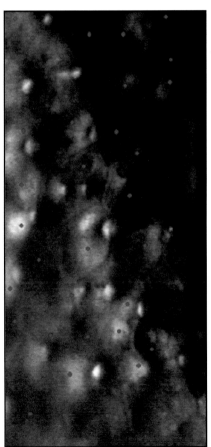

Figure 6-3. Confocal microscopy of endothelial decompensation following cataract surgery in a patient with preoperative Fuchs' dystrophy. The image shows confluent guttae and very few endothelial cells with normal morphology.

Figure 6-4. Confocal microscopy of irido-corneal endothelial syndrome, a disease in which normal corneal endothelial cells are replaced by epithelial-like, migratory cells. The classic finding of "dark-light reversal" of the abnormal endothelial cells shows dark cytoplasm and light cell borders. Light-colored cell nuclei are also visualized within the cytoplasm. (Reprinted with permission from Yvonne Lyons.)

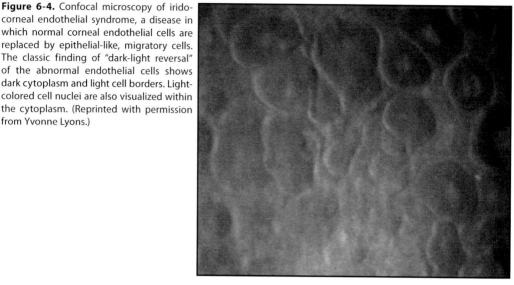

Figure 6-5. Confocal microscopy of suspected Microsporidia organisms (red arrows) in the deep corneal stroma. (Reprinted with permission from Yvonne Lyons.)

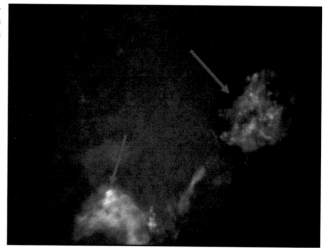

Figure 6-6. Confocal microscopy of fungal keratitis with branching filaments in the mid-corneal stroma. (Reprinted with permission from Yvonne Lyons.)

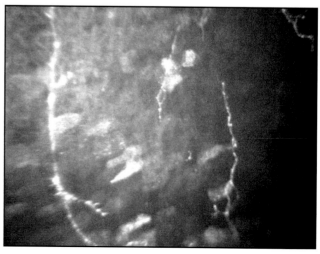

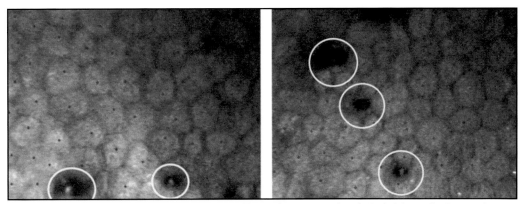

Figure 6-7. Confocal microscopy of the endothelial cell layer of a patient with early Fuchs' dystrophy. Scattered guttae (circled in yellow) appear as hyporeflective spots with occasional central highlights. Note that the surrounding endothelial cells generally maintain uniform shape and size in this mild disease state.

7

ANTERIOR SEGMENT OPTICAL COHERENCE TOMOGRAPHY

C. Maxwell Medert, MD
Hasenin Al-khersan, MD
Ann Q. Tran, MD

Optical coherence tomography (OCT) was initially developed in the 1990s for retinal imaging. The first use of anterior segment OCT (AS-OCT) was reported in 1994 and represented a turning point in anterior segment imaging, which had been previously dominated by ultrasound biomicroscopy (UBM). In principle, AS-OCT uses light waves to form high-resolution, two-dimensional images by measuring the degree of light reflected back from tissues. The imaging modality has had a growing role in ophthalmology, characterizing various pathologies and providing an optical biopsy. Image collection is not technically challenging and no coupling agent is needed with the eye—both of which are limitations for traditional UBM.

AS-OCT has undergone several technical improvements since the 1990s. First, the wavelength has increased from 830 to 1310 nanometers. This change permits deeper tissue penetration so that angle structures and sclera can be better visualized. The shift from time-domain to Fourier-domain to swept-source has allowed for a more rapid acquisition at a higher resolution. Together, these advances have made AS-OCT an invaluable tool in the assessment of anterior pathology of the eye, particularly the cornea.

DIFFERENCES BETWEEN ANTERIOR SEGMENT OPTICAL COHERENCE TOMOGRAPHY AND ULTRASOUND BIOMICROSCOPY

UBM uses ultrasound to visualize structures of the anterior segment. A distinctive advantage of UBM over AS-OCT is the ability to visualize structures posterior to the iris, such as the cili-

Gologorsky D, Rosen RB, eds.
Principles of Ocular Imaging (pp 51-55).
© 2021 Taylor & Francis Group.

ary body. However, UBM is more technically challenging to perform, requiring a skilled operator. While AS-OCT is performed without contact to the patient, UBM requires the use of a probe in a water immersion bath, which can be uncomfortable for the patient. AS-OCT also has a higher resolution than UBM, allowing for detailed imaging of anterior structures. Generally, UBM may be more useful for evaluating the angle, lens, and ciliary body pathology.

HOW TO INTERPRET ANTERIOR SEGMENT OPTICAL COHERENCE TOMOGRAPHY

The primary step in interpreting an AS-OCT is to identify the tissue that has been imaged and understanding the normal anatomy of the cornea and sclera (Figure 7-1). The photographer will usually include a scanning light image with the OCT for orientation. Identifying the depth of a lesion within a particular tissue is the next step. For example, is the lesion epithelial or subepithelial? A benign pterygium will demonstrate subepithelial thickness while ocular surface squamous neoplasia will demonstrate epithelial thickening. The thickness and size of a lesion can be measured and followed over time.

Common terms include the following:

- Reflectivity (hyper vs hypo): a term describing the enhancement ("brightness") of tissues, which is dictated by tissue density

- Thickness: quantitative measurement of tissue/lesion depth

- Transition zone: an abrupt change in the thickness/reflectivity of a tissue layer seen between the border of normal and abnormal tissue

- Epithelial or subepithelial: involvement above or below the corneal and conjunctival epithelium

- Shadowing: area of blockage of normal tissue structures

INDICATIONS OF ANTERIOR SEGMENT OPTICAL COHERENCE TOMOGRAPHY

Like retinal OCT, AS-OCT can be thought of as a cross-sectional "light biopsy" that provides a high resolution image of conjunctival and corneal lesions. AS-OCT is particularly useful for differentiating ocular surface squamous neoplasms from benign lesions. Serial imaging can also be used to monitor lesion size for regression after treatment.

In glaucoma, AS-OCT is also useful as an adjunct to gonioscopy, allowing for visualization of the angle, especially in cases with corneal pathology which limit clinical examination. While this is not the primary indication for AS-OCT, it can be helpful in difficult cases.

Finally, AS-OCT has also been used after Descemet's stripping endothelial keratoplasty and Descemet's membrane endothelial keratoplasty to determine whether or not the graft is attached postoperatively.

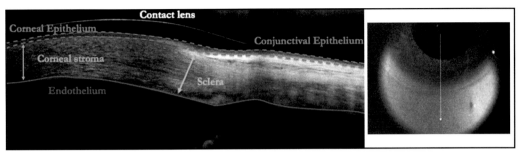

Figure 7-1. Demonstration of the layers of the cornea and sclera on AS-OCT.

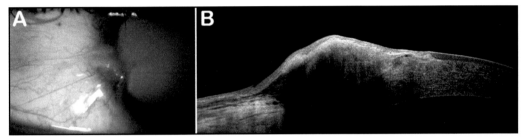

Figure 7-2. (A) Slit lamp photo of a pterygium. (B) Corresponding AS-OCT with subepithelial thickening, shadowing, and hyperreflectivity. The epithelium is preserved without any thickening or hyperreflectivity and lacks a transition point as would be seen with ocular surface neoplasias.

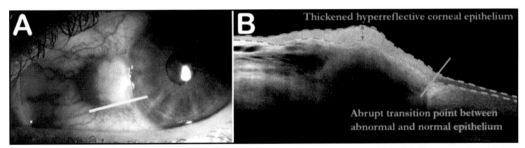

Figure 7-3. (A) Slit lamp photo of a large nodular ocular surface squamous neoplasia. (B) Corresponding AS-OCT with thickened, hyperreflective corneal epithelium with an abrupt transition point. There is shadowing inferior to the corneal epithelium.

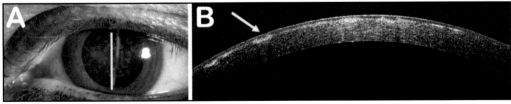

Figure 7-4. (A) Slit lamp photo of granular stromal dystrophy. (B) Corresponding AS-OCT with the arrow highlighting the hyperreflective discrete stromal deposits.

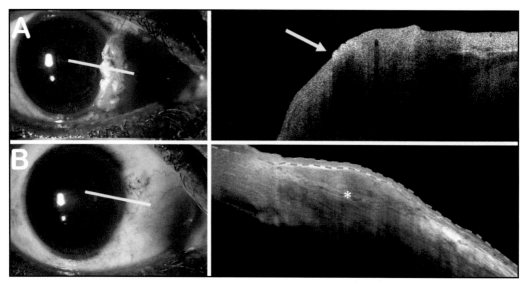

Figure 7-5. (A) Slit lamp photo with corresponding AS-OCT of an irregular ocular surface squamous neoplasia (arrow) with significant shadowing. (B) Slit lamp photograph of the same patient after four cycles of 5-fluorouracil with normalization of corneal epithelium and subepithelial scarring (asterisk).

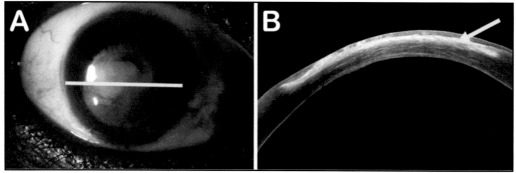

Figure 7-6. (A) Slit lamp photo of a pigmented corneal scar from fungal keratitis. (B) Corresponding AS-OCT with subepithelial stromal hyperreflectivity (arrow) with one-third thickness of the anterior stroma with residual scarring inferiorly, less hyperreflective in nature in the remaining two-thirds of the stroma.

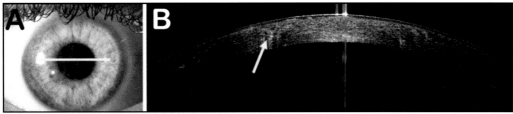

Figure 7-7. (A) Slit lamp photo of lattice corneal dystrophy. (B) Corresponding AS-OCT with the arrow highlighting the amorphous hyperreflective material in the central stroma.

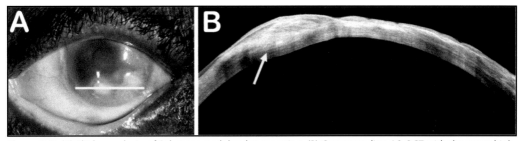

Figure 7-8. (A) Slit lamp photo of Salzmann nodular degeneration. (B) Corresponding AS-OCT with the arrow highlighting the hyperreflective, nodular subepithelial lesion in the stroma.

8

ULTRASOUND BIOMICROSCOPY

Ashwinee Ragam, MD

Ultrasound biomicroscopy (UBM) is a form of high frequency ocular ultrasonography that has been optimized for anterior segment imaging. The transducer direction and probe manipulation are guided by the operator, who is viewing a screen of the real-time image. Compared to conventional A-scan and B-scan ultrasonography which operate at lower frequencies (10 to 20 MHz) for posterior segment imaging, UBM employs higher frequencies (35 to 100 MHz) that provide the finer resolution necessary to discriminate delicate anterior segment structures. UBM requires a coupling medium between the oscillating ultrasound probe and the ocular surface. This can be accomplished using a probe cover filled with distilled water or with an open soft plastic shell placed between the eyelids, filled with methylcellulose, in a supine patient.

In an anatomically normal eye, UBM can be used to image the cornea, anterior chamber, scleral spur, iris, ciliary body, posterior chamber, and anterior lens surface. UBM can also be used to perform white-to-white, sulcus-to-sulcus, and anterior chamber depth measurements, which may be needed for cataract and refractive procedures.

UBM devices vary in their specifications. The image resolution and depth produced by a particular machine are dependent on its ultrasound probe frequency, the ratio of the focal length to the transducer diameter, and the duration of the pulse. Higher frequencies and shorter focal lengths result in higher resolution images, but poorer penetration (ie, the ultrasound can generate sharp images of the cornea, but cannot demonstrate deeper structures).

Gologorsky D, Rosen RB, eds.
Principles of Ocular Imaging (pp 57-60).
© 2021 Taylor & Francis Group.

UBM and anterior segment optical coherence tomography (AS-OCT) are distinct modalities for imaging the anterior segment. AS-OCT is advantageous over UBM in that its non-contact technique is more comfortable for patients, it acquires images more quickly without the need of an experienced operator, and it provides better resolution of more anterior structures such as the cornea. However, UBM is superior at visualizing structures posterior to the iris, which makes it invaluable in evaluating conditions like angle-closure glaucoma (such as pupillary block and plateau iris) and pathology of the ciliary body (such as cysts, clefts, and tumors).

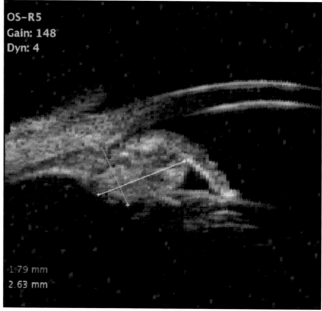

Figure 8-1. UBM image of a ciliary body melanoma with measured dimensions in millimeters. The mass is pushing the iris anteriorly, which leads to angle closure.

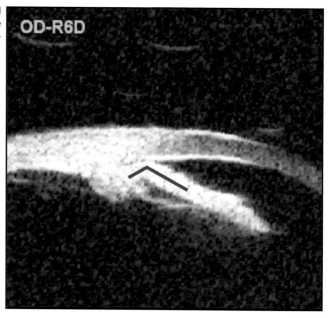

Figure 8-2. UBM image of plateau iris and a narrow anterior chamber angle. The blue line traces iridocorneal touch and the plateau iris configuration.

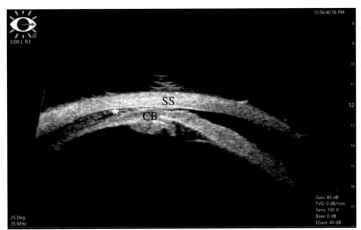

Figure 8-3. UBM image of a cyclodialysis cleft. The fluid-filled suprachoroidal space (asterisk) results from separation between the scleral spur (SS) and ciliary body (CB).

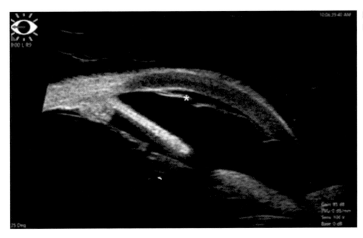

Figure 8-4. UBM image of a Descemet's detachment (asterisk).

Figure 8-5. UBM image of a pseudophakic eye with otherwise normal anterior segment structures. (A) Cornea. (B) Anterior chamber. (C) Iris. (D) Posterior chamber. (E) Intraocular lens in the capsular bag. (F) Ciliary body. (G) Sclera. Asterisk: Scleral spur. Arrow: Open anterior chamber angle.

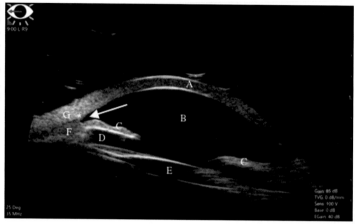

Figure 8-6. UBM image of a ciliary body cyst with measured dimensions in millimeters.

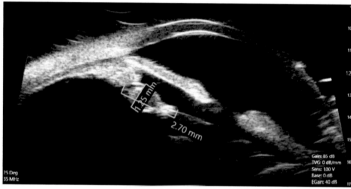

9

Biometry for Intraocular Lens Calculations

Ashwinee Ragam, MD

Biometry, the general term defining a method of applying mathematics to biological sciences, is used in ophthalmology to indicate measurement of the size and shape of the eye and perform intraocular lens (IOL) calculations. Determining the IOL power to be implanted during cataract surgery requires measuring or identifying several variables: the eye's axial length, average corneal power, and anterior chamber depth; A-constant of the chosen IOL; and target postoperative refraction. Axial length is measured as the distance from the anterior pole to the posterior pole of the eye.

The original regression formula (known as SRK) for calculating the power (P) of an IOL uses the following equation: $P = A - 0.9K - 2.5L$. A stands for the A-constant specific to the chosen IOL; K represents the average corneal curvature; and L equals axial length. The SRK formula is now obsolete and has been replaced by newer theoretical formulas which account for long and short eyes, and effective lens position. Regardless of the formula used, a 1 mm change in axial length translates to a 2.5 to 3 diopter (D) change in IOL power, so precise measurements are critical. Axial lengths differing by more than 0.3 mm between two otherwise normal eyes of a single patient should be remeasured to ensure accuracy.

Gologorsky D, Rosen RB, eds.
Principles of Ocular Imaging (pp 61-67).
© 2021 Taylor & Francis Group.

Ultrasound Biometry

Ultrasound (A-scan) biometry is the original modality for measuring the axial length of an eye. The ultrasound probe can either make direct contact with the patient's cornea or use an immersion bath as a coupling medium. Sound waves generated by the ultrasound probe travel from the anterior corneal vertex and through the eye, along a path independent of patient fixation, striking various interfaces of intraocular structures. The beams are broad and terminate somewhere near the center of the macula at the internal limiting membrane. Returning echoes of intraocular structures are received by the probe tip and converted into spikes that are then displayed on the screen.

The greater the density difference at the acoustic interface of an intraocular structure, the larger the spike produced. Contact A-scans should produce five high-amplitude spikes from a normal phakic eye: the probe tip-cornea interface, anterior lens capsule, posterior lens capsule, retina, and sclera. Immersion A-scans produce one initial spike for the probe tip-bath interface and read the anterior and posterior cornea as two close but separate spikes, therefore displaying seven high-amplitude spikes in total. Poor retinal spikes (ie, not sharply rising at a 90-degree angle) may indicate that the probe is not perpendicular to the macula or that there is a macular pathology. Poor or absent scleral spikes may indicate that the beam is aligned with the optic nerve instead of the macula.

The ultrasound velocity should be adjusted based on the patient's lens status (eg, phakic, pseudophakic, aphakic) as the speed of sound changes with media density. Very dense cataracts can absorb passing sound waves, so most machines have a dense cataract setting to compensate for this. The examiner may also need to increase the machine's gain, or amplification of the echoes, to obtain adequate spikes.

The distance between the anterior corneal and retinal spikes gives the axial length of the eye. Contact A-scans often cause compression of the cornea, which can falsely decrease the axial length and reduce scan reproducibility. The immersion technique eliminates the compression variable and allows for more consistent readings, and is thus considered the gold standard for ultrasonic axial length measurement.

For a single measured eye, the axial length and anterior chamber diameter are reported as the average of multiple A-scan readings. The examiner should only include 5 to 10 of the most consistent readings—deleting the outliers—and aim for a standard deviation of less than 0.10 mm.

Optical Biometry

Unlike ultrasound biometry, optical biometry employs light waves that have shorter wavelengths and produce higher resolution images than sound waves. Using the principle of partial coherence interferometry, dual beams of infrared light are emitted by a diode laser, passed from the corneal vertex to the retinal pigment epithelium of the fovea, and then reflected back. The interference patterns of the signals returned are analyzed to calculate the length of the eye. The path that the light travels is dependent on patient fixation; therefore, optical biometry measures axial length along the true visual axis. The non-contact technique of optical biometry offers advantages over ultrasound biometry including enhanced patient comfort, reduced operator variability, and lack of corneal compression. The reproducibility of axial length and anterior chamber depth measurements are much higher in optical biometry. However, its utility is limited in eyes with media opacities (eg, corneal scar, posterior subcapsular or very dense nuclear cataract, vitreous hemorrhage) through which the passing of light waves and patient fixation are impeded.

Modern optical biometers can also measure anterior corneal curvature, corneal thickness, lens thickness, and horizontal white-to-white diameter. When a single machine can perform both axial length and keratometry measurements, it can subsequently calculate IOL powers for multiple A-constants, at several target refractions, using different IOL formulae. Newer generation optical biometers have a topography function which can assist in planning for a toric IOL implantation.

The IOLMaster (Carl Zeiss Meditec, Inc) was FDA approved in the United States in 2000 and is the first optical biometry device to be widely used in ophthalmology practice. The waveform graph of a normal eye should show a central, tall, thin primary spike (known as the *primary maxima*) surrounded by a set of shorter secondary maxima, within a horizontal line of background "static." The IOLMaster requires examiners to obtain at least five scans/eye, which are then combined to produce a composite waveform graph and single-axial length measurement. Individual scans should not differ by more than 0.05 mm in axial length measurement to ensure consistent readings. The signal-to-noise ratio (SNR) reports the overall scan quality; the threshold for a sufficient SNR is 2.0, but examiners should aim for greater than 10.0. Scan settings should be adjusted based on lens status (eg, phakic, aphakic, pseudophakic) and for the presence of silicone oil. For keratometry readings, the IOLMaster reflects six points of light, arranged in a 2.3- to 2.5-mm diameter hexagon, off of the air-tear film interface.

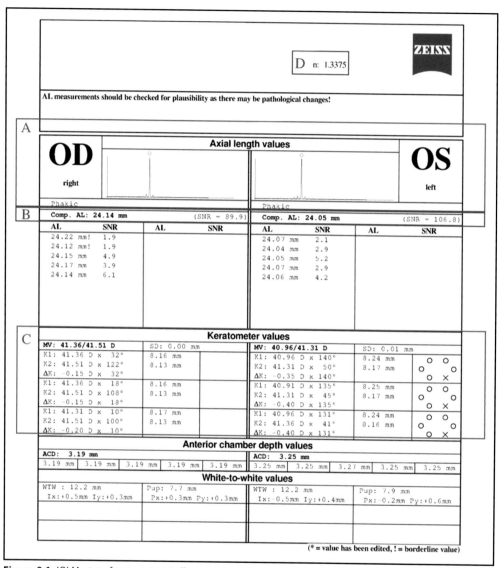

Figure 9-1. IOLMaster of two anatomically normal, phakic eyes from a single patient. (A) The axial length (AL) waveforms of each eye show a well-defined primary maximum surrounded by smaller secondary maxima; there is little to no background "static." (B) There is less than a 0.3-mm difference between the composite axial lengths of the two eyes and the overall SNR in each eye, which is considered acceptable. (C) Keratometry measurements show average flat and steep corneal curvatures based on three readings in each eye. (D) A refractive index of 1.3375 is used for calculating corneal power.

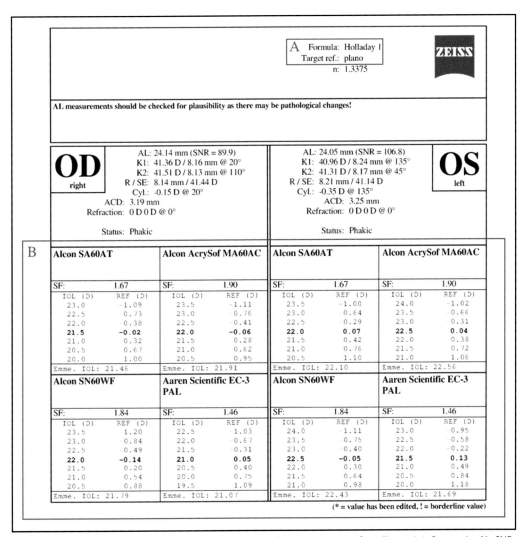

Figure 9-2. Another view of the IOLMaster measurements of the same patient from Figure 9-1. Composite AL, SNR, magnitude and meridian of flat corneal curvature (K1), magnitude and meridian of steep corneal curvature (K2), average corneal curvature (R/SE), central corneal astigmatism (Cyl), and anterior chamber depth (ACD) are displayed for each eye. The Holladay formula (A) is used to calculate the powers (B) of different intraocular lens models and their expected postoperative refractions, ranging around the inputted target refraction (plano). Keratometry values measured from the IOLMaster are used to perform lens power calculations.

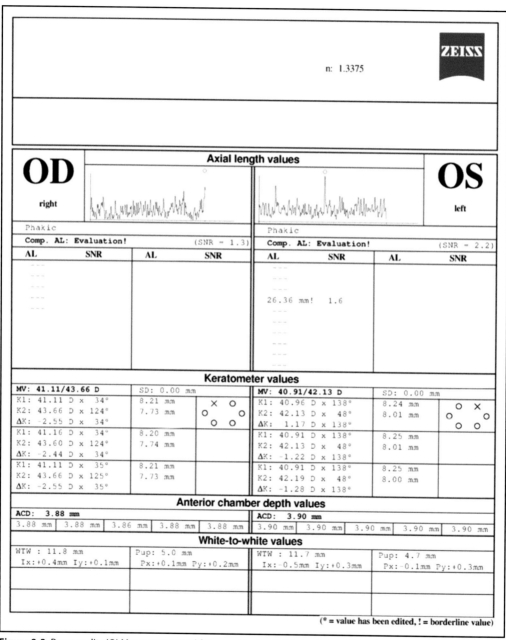

Axial length values			
OD right			**OS** left

Phakic

Comp. AL: Evaluation!		(SNR = 1.3)	Comp. AL: Evaluation!		(SNR = 2.2)
AL	**SNR**	**AL**	**AL**	**SNR**	**AL**

AL	SNR	AL	SNR	AL	SNR	AL	SNR
- - -				- - -			
- - -				- - -			
- - -				26.36 mm!	1.6		
- - -				- - -			
- - -				- - -			
				- - -			
				- - -			
				- - -			
				- - -			

Keratometer values

MV: 41.11/43.66 D		SD: 0.00 mm	MV: 40.91/42.13 D		SD: 0.00 mm
K1: 41.11 D x 34°	8.21 mm	✕ ○	K1: 40.96 D x 138°	8.24 mm	○ ✕
K2: 43.66 D x 124°	7.73 mm	○ ○	K2: 42.13 D x 48°	8.01 mm	○ ○
ΔK: -2.55 D x 34°		○ ○	ΔK: 1.17 D x 138°		○ ○
K1: 41.16 D x 34°	8.20 mm		K1: 40.91 D x 138°	8.25 mm	
K2: 43.60 D x 124°	7.74 mm		K2: 42.13 D x 48°	8.01 mm	
ΔK: -2.44 D x 34°			ΔK: -1.22 D x 138°		
K1: 41.11 D x 35°	8.21 mm		K1: 40.91 D x 138°	8.25 mm	
K2: 43.66 D x 125°	7.73 mm		K2: 42.19 D x 48°	8.00 mm	
ΔK: -2.55 D x 35°			ΔK: -1.28 D x 138°		

Anterior chamber depth values

ACD: 3.88 mm					ACD: 3.90 mm				
3.88 mm	3.88 mm	3.86 mm	3.88 mm	3.88 mm	3.90 mm	3.90 mm	3.90 mm	3.90 mm	3.90 mm

White-to-white values

WTW : 11.8 mm	Pup: 5.0 mm	WTW : 11.7 mm	Pup: 4.7 mm
Ix:+0.4mm Iy:+0.1mm	Px:+0.1mm Py:+0.2mm	Ix:-0.5mm Iy:+0.3mm	Px:-0.1mm Py:+0.3mm

(* = value has been edited, ! = borderline value)

Figure 9-3. Poor-quality IOLMaster generated from a patient with bilateral posterior subcapsular cataracts. Note that the AL waveform of each eye displays significant noise without the definitive spikes expected of a normal phakic scan. AL measurements are unable to be generated from this scan. Even though the composite SNR in the left eye is >2.0, the waveform alone should be enough to warn the examiner of the low utility of this scan.

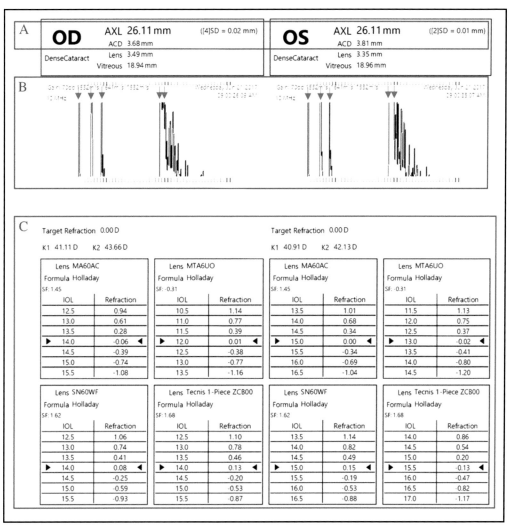

Figure 9-4. Contact A-scan ultrasound of two anatomically normal, phakic eyes from a single patient. (A) Average AL measurement for each eye with the number of readings averaged in brackets and standard deviation (SD) in millimeters. (B) Five normal high-amplitude spikes produced from each eye are indicated with arrows. (C) The Holladay formula is used to calculate the power of different intraocular lens models and their expected postoperative refractions, ranging around the inputted target refraction (0.00 D). Keratometry values were measured using a separate modality and manually entered in order to perform lens power calculations.

Section III
Retina

Section Editors

Daniel Gologorsky, MD, MBA

Richard B. Rosen, MD

10

FUNDUS PHOTOGRAPHY

Daniel Gologorsky, MD, MBA

The purpose of fundus photography is to establish a visual record of the posterior segment. It can be an invaluable visual adjunct to the documented record in providing an objective narrative of the patient's physical examination at any given moment in time. In the clinical setting, serial fundus photography is especially helpful when comparing fundoscopic changes over time, especially when assessing subtle interval changes in diabetic or glaucomatous eyes.

In the past, fundus photography was limited by insufficient light, long exposures, eye motion artifacts, and prominent corneal reflexes. Over the last several decades, fundus photographic systems have improved dramatically with advances such as electronic illumination control, pupil tracking, non-mydriatic imaging, high-resolution digital image capture, widefield imaging, and most recently, portability.

A fundus camera is comprised of a specialized low-power telescope with an attached camera. The optical design of the fundus camera is similar to that of an indirect ophthalmoscope in that the observation and illumination systems follow parallel paths, allowing for the capture of crisp and clear images. A fundus camera provides an upright and magnified view of the retina. A standard camera provides a 30-degree angle of retinal view with 2.5x image magnification. Keep in mind that although the angle of view can be modified, magnification will respond in an inverse manner. Ultra-wide field imaging can now capture more than 200 degrees of the retina, covering over 80% of the tissue in a single view.

In contrast to color fundus photography, where the retina is illuminated by white light, red-free fundus photography utilizes a green filter in absorbing the overwhelming red wavelengths of light which are reflected from the retina. This enhances the contrast of retinal structures and pathologies, darkening hemorrhages, highlighting drusen and exudates, and reveals the superficial details of nerve fiber layer defects and epiretinal membranes. Red-free photography is typically included as the initial baseline photo prior to a fluorescein angiography sequence.

Gologorsky D, Rosen RB, eds.
Principles of Ocular Imaging (pp 71-80).
© 2021 Taylor & Francis Group.

A recent alternative to traditional color digital-fundus photography is confocal scanning laser ophthalmoscopy, a technology that uses a near-infrared diode laser beam, rather than a bright flash of white light, to illuminate the retina. The laser requires a lower level of light exposure at a nearly invisible wavelength, which improves patient comfort, as it rapidly scans the posterior pole at a high frame rate and at high magnification. Although not in color, the images produced by this monochromatic laser system are finely detailed with high contrast with more nuanced structural delineation than those with standard fundus cameras.

Fundus photographic systems have become more portable and have evolved into handheld systems, allowing for their meaningful use for screening purposes by primary care physicians, emergency room staff, or health care workers in the field. Furthermore, with the advent and proliferation of smartphones, handheld adaptors that complement mobile applications allow for rapid fundus photography; although, these systems are limited by their central view only, making them most useful for macular pathology.

Figure 10-1. Fundus photo of the right eye taken with a traditional fundus camera. The fundus does not demonstrate any obvious pathology.

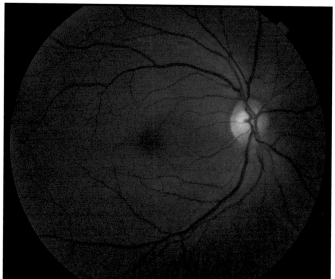

Figure 10-2. Fundus photo demonstrating congenital hypertrophy of the retinal pigment epithelium with an adjacent horseshoe tear that was recently surrounded with laser treatment.

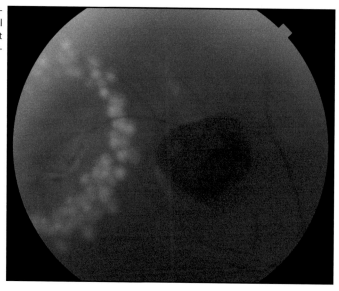

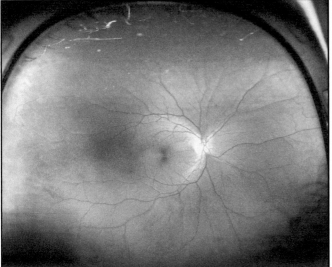

Figure 10-3. Widefield fundus photo taken with a widefield Optos (Nikon) camera. The fundus does not demonstrate any obvious pathology.

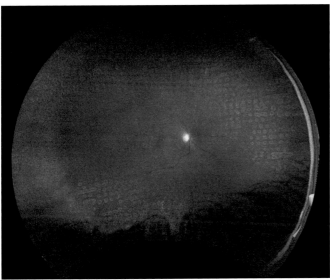

Figure 10-4. Widefield fundus photo demonstrating proliferative diabetic retinopathy treated with copious panretinal photocoagulation.

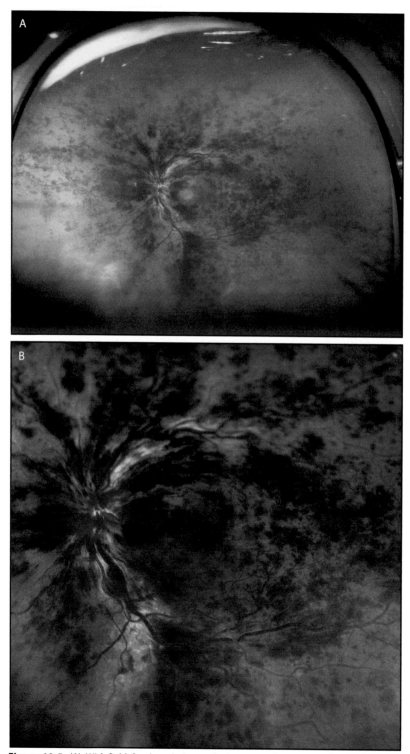

Figure 10-5. (A) Widefield fundus photograph demonstrating a central retinal venous occlusion of the left eye. (B) Note the striking optic nerve head edema, vascular tortuosity, macular edema, and intraretinal hemorrhages.

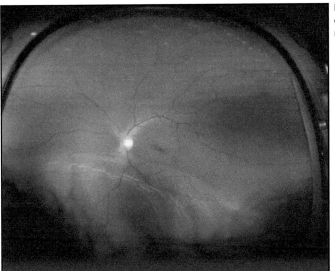

Figure 10-6. Widefield fundus photo demonstrating an inferior retinal detachment.

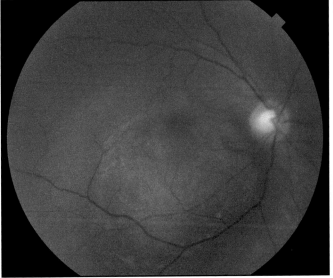

Figure 10-7. Fundus photo demonstrating a large peripapillary choroidal melanoma in the macula. Note the orange pigment overlaying the surface of the mass.

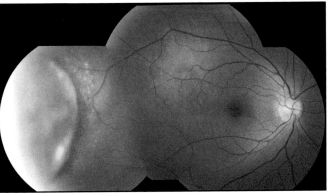

Figure 10-8. Montage fundus photo taken in order to capture the temporal choroidal mass.

Figure 10-9. Fundus photo of a patient with exudative age-related macular degeneration demonstrating macular drusen with a choroidal neovascular membrane associated with hemorrhage.

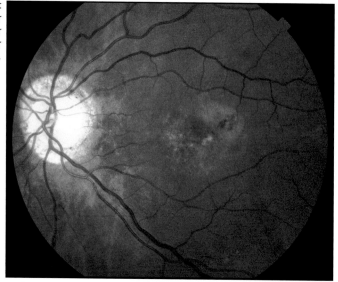

Figure 10-10. Fundus photo demonstrating geographic atrophy in a patient with advanced nonexudative ("dry") macular degeneration. The atrophy unmasks the underlying choroidal vasculature.

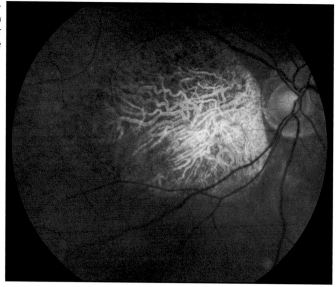

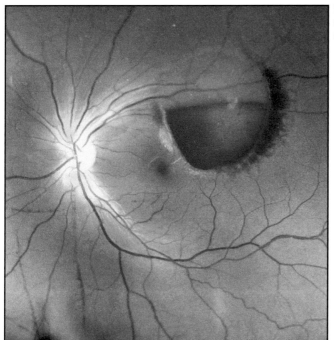

Figure 10-11. Fundus photograph demonstrating a classic scaphoid, or "boat-shaped," preretinal hemorrhage.

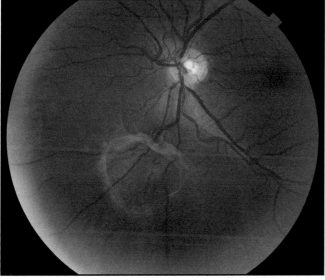

Figure 10-12. A fundus photograph showing a traumatic posterior vitreous detachment in a teenager. The detached garland of peripapillary tissue (ie, Weiss ring) is seen floating in front of the retina down below the center of the image.

Figure 10-13. A fundus photograph demonstrating a submacular hemorrhage in an older patient. Vision loss was severe.

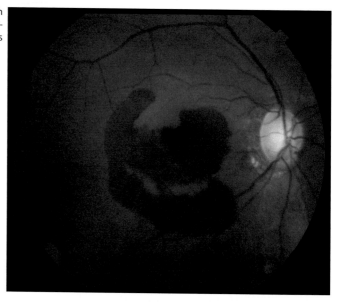

Figure 10-14. Widefield fundus photo showing multiple horseshoe tears that had been previously surrounded by laser.

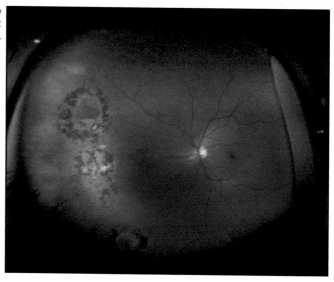

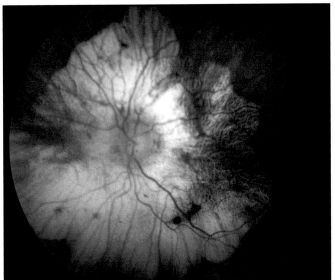

Figure 10-15. Color fundus photo showing staphylomatous changes to a highly myopic eye, with peripapillary atrophy and geographic atrophy.

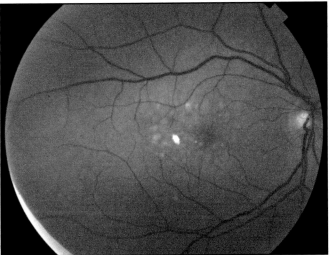

Figure 10-16. Red-free fundus photo demonstrating calcified drusen in the macula. Note the "light-colored" optic nerve of red-free photos that distinguish these images from autofluorescence photos marked by a "dark-colored" optic nerve.

Figure 10-17. Smartphone fundus photography enabled with the aid of a 20-D condensing lens holder reveals an intraocular foreign body lying on the retina. (Reprinted with permission from Michael Jansen, MD.)

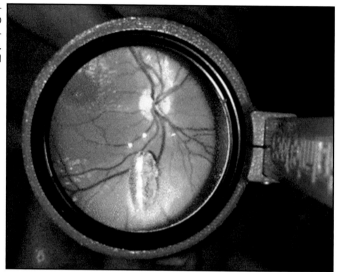

Figure 10-18. Smartphone fundus photography using a handheld 20-D condensing lens (without an adaptor) demonstrates a preretinal hemorrhage.

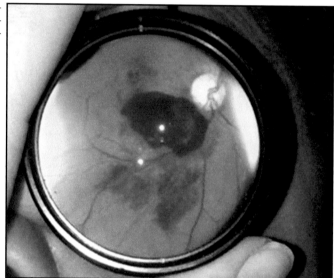

11

Fluorescein Angiography

Daniel Gologorsky, MD, MBA

Fluorescein angiography (FA) was first described by two medical students, Novotny and Alvis, in 1961. It was subsequently adopted universally among ophthalmologists as the foundation for retinal diagnostics. FA entails the intravenous injection of sodium fluorescein dye into the peripheral circulation with subsequent photographic capture as the dye courses through the retinal circulation. FA can reveal important retinal pathology and is most commonly used in the context of vascular diseases of the retina and choroid, such as diabetic retinopathy and vascular occlusive disease.

The FA procedure involves injecting a bolus of fluorescein sodium into a hand or arm vein, commonly the antecubital. Approximately 80% of the dye molecules bind to plasma proteins, principally albumin, leaving the remaining 20% of unbound molecules available to fluoresce when excited by light, and ultimately be imaged. This process, *fluorescence*, refers to the ability of a molecule to absorb a photon of one wavelength and then emit a photon of a different wavelength. In this case, fluorescein absorbs blue light (465 to 490 nanometers [nm]), and as the excited molecule returns to its ground state, it emits a photon of lower energy (and longer wavelength) in the form of yellow-green light (520 to 530 nm). A specialized fundus camera, equipped with a matched pair of exciter and barrier filters within these precise wavelength ranges, captures only emitted light through the barrier filter and records the angiographic sequence. A timer annotates each frame of the study.

As an alternative to the traditional fundus camera, confocal scanning laser ophthalmoscopy (cSLO) have also been used to capture FAs. These instruments use a laser beam of the appropriate excitation wavelength to scan across the fundus in a raster pattern illuminating successive elements of the retina, point-by-point. The confocal optical system and laser illumination combine to produce high contrast, finely detailed images, and can capture crisp angiograms.

Gologorsky D, Rosen RB, eds.
Principles of Ocular Imaging (pp 81-92).
© 2021 Taylor & Francis Group.

Once circulated throughout the body, fluorescein is metabolized by both the liver and kidneys and is ultimately eliminated through the urine within 24 to 36 hours of administration. Patients can expect a slightly yellow skin hue or tanned appearance for several hours and an orange discoloration of the urine for up to several days after the procedure. While typically safe and unremarkable for over 90% of patients, there are some important side effects that need to be mentioned to the patient. The most common side effects are mild and self limited, and include transient nausea (infrequently leading to vomiting) occurring minutes immediately following injection. Moderate reactions affecting less than 2% of FA patients include allergic pruritus and urticaria that typically responds to antihistamines. Severe reactions, including anaphylaxis, laryngeal edema, bronchospasm, seizures, and cardiac arrest are exceedingly rare and occur in less than 1 in 100,000 patients undergoing FA.

The angiographic sequence of a typical fluorescein study is marked by several phases of the ocular circulation that have been classically described. These include the choroidal, arterial, arterial-venous (capillary), early venous, late venous, and recirculation phases. Average time for the fluorescein bolus to circulate from the antecubital vein of the arm to the retina is 10 to 12 seconds. The choroidal phase is marked by a patchy or geographic map-like filling pattern of the choriocapillaris. It is challenging to study the choroidal circulation with a FA as dye rapidly leaks from these vessels and the retinal pigment epithelium (RPE) acts as a translucent screen, diffusing the view. During the choroidal phase, any cilioretinal arteries present will also fill. The arterial phase (11 to 14 seconds) commences once the dye circulates to the central retinal artery and its branches. During this time, the retinal arteries light up while the veins remain dark. Shortly thereafter, the capillary phase (or the arterio-venous phase) occurs, briefly highlighting the perifoveal capillary network. The early venous phase (13 to 20 seconds) is marked by the distinctive fluorescein filling of the retinal veins through laminar flow, where dye lining the walls of the veins appears before their lumens fill with dye. The late venous phase is marked by a notable hyperfluorescence of the entire retinal vasculature system. The recirculation phase takes place during the 5 to 10 minutes following the fluorescein injection. At this point in time no tissue should fluoresce except of the optic disc and scar tissue.

There are various reasons tissue might hyperfluoresce in FA, both normal and pathologic. *Normal autofluorescence* occurs when certain tissue spontaneously produces fluorescent light when stimulated by light containing blue wavelengths. Optic nerve head drusen and astrocytic hamartomas are two tissues that classically demonstrate autofluorescence. Taking fundus photographs with a barrier filter in place prior to the injection of fluorescein can be helpful in identifying autofluorescent tissues and distinguishing them from pathologic hyperfluorescence.

Abnormal hyperfluorescence typically occurs in four patterns:

1. *Window defects* result from abnormal transmission of normal choroidal fluorescence through a defect in the RPE. This defect in the RPE screen essentially unmasks the choroidal signal normally hidden beneath the RPE. Geographic atrophy is a classic example of a lesion that exhibits window defect hyperfluorescence, but window defect can occur due to any RPE degenerative process. Hyperfluorescence from a window defect is usually more prominent early in the FA and declines with time corresponding to the decreasing concentration of dye in the choroid.

2. *Leakage* describes fluorescein dye that escapes the intravascular space. Leakage is typically seen as a small spot of hyperfluorescent in an early frame that increases in size and intensity as the angiogram progresses, corresponding to the escape of dye from leaking blood vessels. Leakage is most commonly encountered in the setting of retinal neovascularization secondary to proliferative diabetic disease, diabetic macular edema, choroidal neovascular vessels, or venous occlusive events.

3. *Pooling* refers to the accumulation of fluorescein in a cavity with defined borders. The angiogram is marked by hyperfluorescence that appears early, and increases in intensity (similar to leakage), but does not extend beyond the boundaries of its cavity. Examples of leakage include microaneurysms, pigment epithelial detachment, retinal arterial macroaneurysm, and cystoid edema.

4. *Staining* refers to the uptake of fluorescein into structures such as drusen, the optic disc, peripapillary atrophy, or scar tissue. Staining causes hyperfluorescence that gradually increases in intensity throughout the FA, but without an increase in the area of hyperfluorescence over time. Unlike a window defect, staining maintains hyperfluorescence late in the FA.

Abnormal hypofluorescence typically occurs in two patterns:

1. *Blocking* refers to the masking of normal fluorescence of retinal structures. This can be due to lens opacity, vitreous hemorrhage, preretinal hemorrhage, intraretinal hemorrhage, subretinal hemorrhage, or pigmentary changes. Choroidal fluorescence can also be blocked by nevi, melanomas, or lipofuscin (as in the "dark choroid" of Stargardt's disease).

2. *Filling defect* is an area or vessel lacking in fluorescence due to perfusion blockage in the setting of arterial or venous occlusion. Capillary nonperfusion refers to such areas that frequently result of advanced diabetic retinopathy.

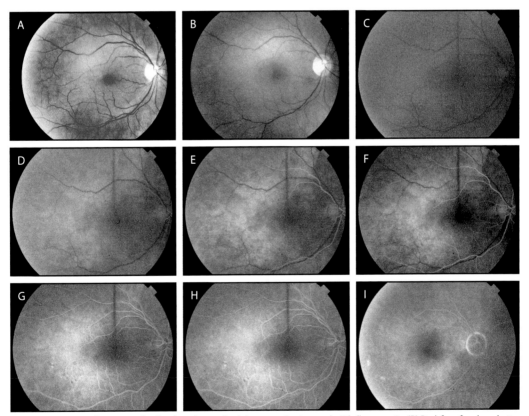

Figure 11-1. Normal FA. (A) Color fundus photo of a right eye to be imaged with fluorescein. (B) Red-free fundus photo. (C) Pre-injection view. After injection, imaging captures the (D) choroidal phase, (E) early arterial phase, (F) early laminar phase, (G) early venous phase, (H) full venous phase, and (I) late recirculation phase.

Figure 11-2. Proliferative diabetic retinopathy with pooling (microaneurysms),
leaking (neovascularization), blocking (preretinal hemorrhage), and filling
defect (capillary dropout).

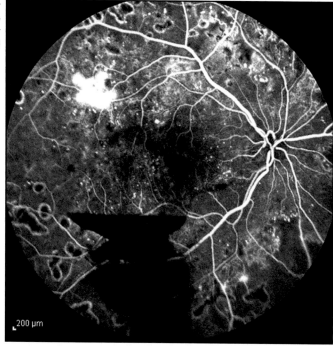

Figure 11-3. Proliferative diabetic retinopathy with significant leakage due to
neovascularization. Note the peripheral
staining due to scars from prior panretinal photocoagulation (PRP) treatment.

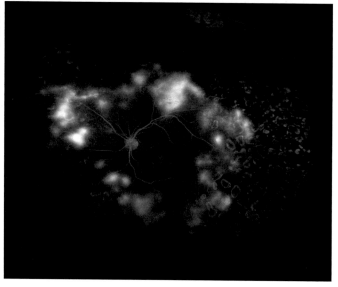

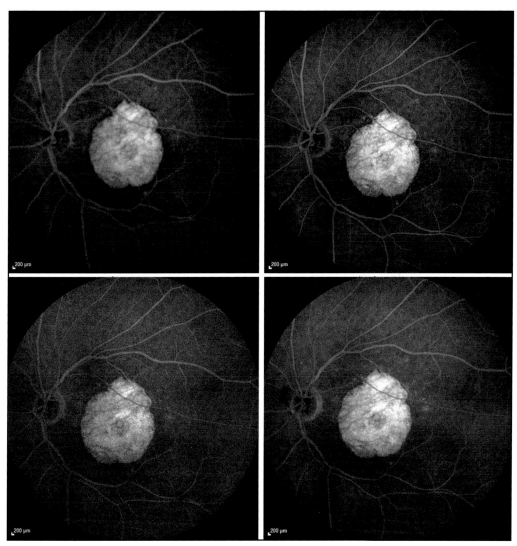

Figure 11-4. Nonexudative age-related macular degeneration with geographic atrophy demonstrating window defect.

Figure 11-5. Sea fan neovascularization with temporal leakage in a patient with sickle-cell retinopathy.

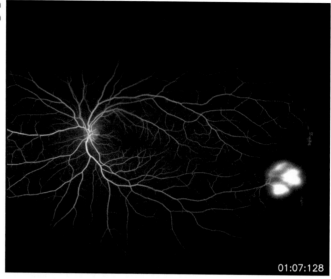

Figure 11-6. Central retinal venous occlusion demonstrating hyperfluorescent leakage and hypofluorescent blockage from hemorrhage and vascular nonperfusion.

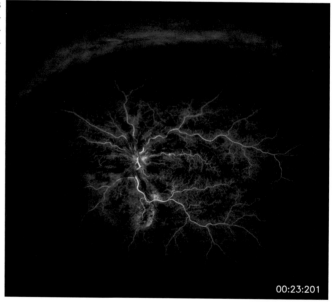

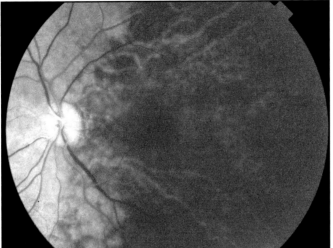

Figure 11-7. Central retinal artery occlusion showing global hypofluorescence (with the exception of optic nerve vasculature) and the lack of a cilioretinal artery in a patient with giant cell arteritis.

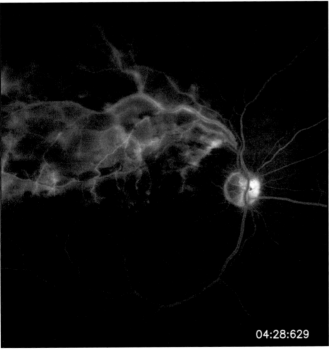

Figure 11-8. Superior branch retinal artery occlusion with leakage and delayed filling.

Figure 11-9. An early frame (52 seconds) showing an old branch retinal vein occlusion with notable nonperfusion in the distribution of the temporal macula and periphery.

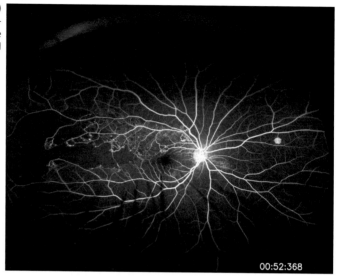

Figure 11-10. Late frame (5 minutes) of the same branch retinal vein occlusion demonstrating neovascularization on the border of perfused and nonperfused tissue.

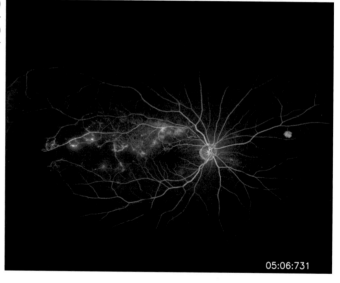

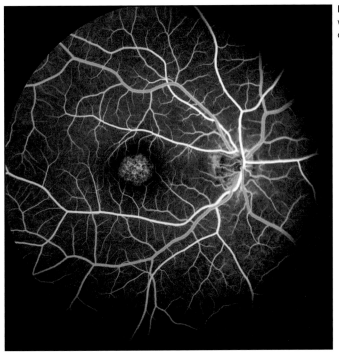

Figure 11-11. Window defect in a patient with bilateral "bull's eye" maculopathy due to a retinal pigment epitheliopathy.

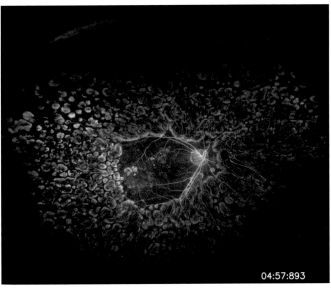

Figure 11-12. A patient with proliferative diabetic retinopathy treated with extensive PRP. FA does not show any active neovascularization. Note the staining of the PRP scars.

Figure 11-13. Exudative age-related macular degeneration with a new choroidal neovascular membrane (hyperfluorescent spot) causing significant subretinal hemorrhage (hypofluorescent blocking).

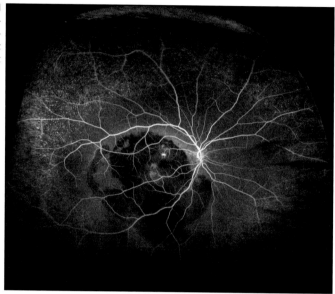

Figure 11-14. Choroidal melanoma with leaking foci. The classic double circulation pattern is not evident here.

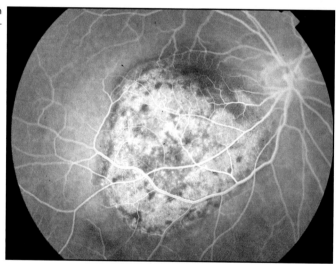

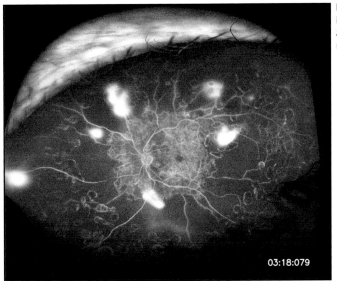

Figure 11-15. A profoundly ischemic retina with large areas of capillary dropout and clouds of focal leakage due to active neovascular vessels.

03:18:079

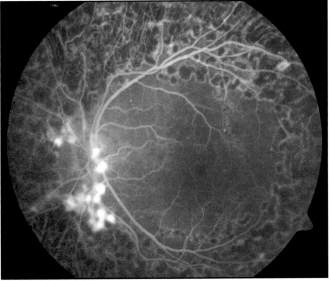

Figure 11-16. Leakage due to neovascularization of the disc in a patient with proliferative diabetic retinopathy treated previously with PRP.

Figure 11-17. Chronic central serous retinopathy showing (A) multiple areas of staining within the RPE and two focal "hot spots." Another case of chronic central serous retinopathy demonstrating (B) a "runoff" or "guttering" phenomenon.

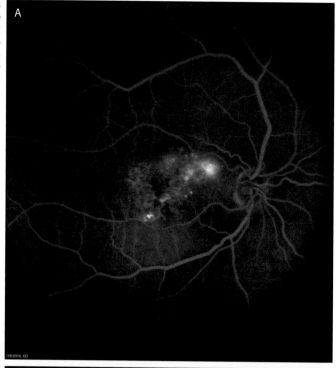

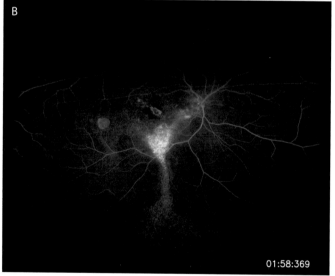

12

INDOCYANINE GREEN ANGIOGRAPHY

Daniel Gologorsky, MD, MBA

The choroid lies between the sclera and the retina and its details are largely obscured by the retinal pigment epithelium (RPE). The visible wavelengths of light emitted by fluorescein are limited in their ability to reveal choroidal pathology. Indocyanine green (ICG), however, emits wavelengths of light in the near infrared range, enabling deeper tissue penetration and allowing for a meaningful evaluation of choroidal circulation by the clinician. ICG is often utilized to elucidate choroidal pathology such as occult choroidal neovascularization (CNV) or choroiditis.

ICG is administered intravenously at a typical dose of 25 mg, often sequentially following fluorescein injection, or mixed together in one dye mixture. ICG angiography is a relatively safe procedure with less frequent transient nausea and vomiting than fluorescein angiography. Life threatening anaphylactic reactions are exceedingly rare. ICG dyes contain iodide, and as such, are contraindicated for patients with iodide or shellfish allergies. ICG is metabolized hepatically, and so should be avoided in those taking metformin or with liver disease.

The near-infrared fluorescence of ICG allows it to be more visible through blood, lipid, fluid, and pigment compared to fluorescein. Over 98% of ICG molecules bind to plasma proteins, as opposed to 80% of fluorescein molecules. The higher plasma protein binding limits the molecules that are available to leak through choroidal capillary fenestrations, enhancing the definition of choroidal vasculature and CNV.

During the early phase of ICG angiography, 1 minute after injecting the dye, large choroidal arteries and veins are highlighted. The middle phase commences 5 to 15 minutes after injection, at which point the choroidal vasculature become less distinct and more diffuse, and a homogeneous choroidal fluorescence is observed. At this time, any hyperfluorescent lesions appear bright against the fading background. CNV are best detected in the late phase, during which a hyperfluorescent

Gologorsky D, Rosen RB, eds.
Principles of Ocular Imaging (pp 93-98).
© 2021 Taylor & Francis Group.

lesion is visible against a darker background. Poorly defined or occult CNV appear stained by the ICG dye during the late phase. Note that ICG angiography is best suited for poorly defined or occult CNV; well-defined or classic CNV have a variable appearance on ICG angiography.

In terms of nomenclature, a "hot spot" refers to a focal area of an occult CNV that is less than 1 disc diameter in size and is well delineated. If the hyperfluorescent lesion exceeds 1 disc diameter, then the lesion demonstrates "placoid" hyperfluorescence.

Figure 12-1. ICG angiography of a polypoidal choroidal vasculopathy lesion demonstrating macular hyperfluorescence.

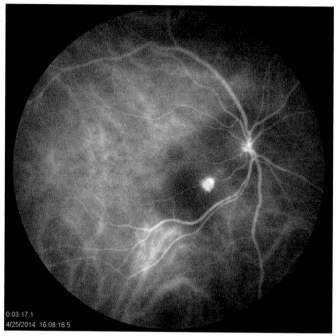

Figure 12-2. An early-phase ICG angiogram demonstrating fine macular telangiectasia of the left macula.

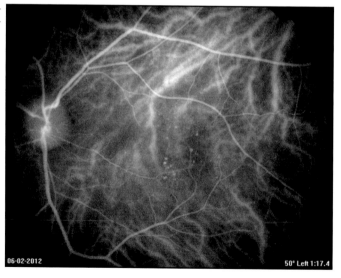

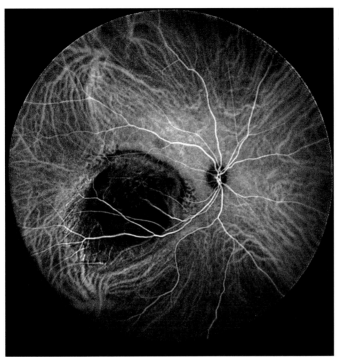

Figure 12-3. ICG angiography of the right eye of a 27-year-old woman demonstrating hypofluorescence in the distribution of a choroidal tumor.

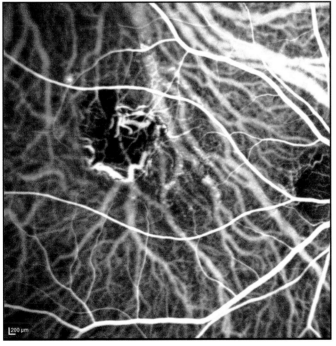

Figure 12-4. An early phase ICG angiography image of the right eye of a 66-year-old woman with a clearly delineated choroidal neovascular membrane.

Figure 12-5. Late-phase ICG angiography of the left eye of a 59-year-old man with angioid streaks.

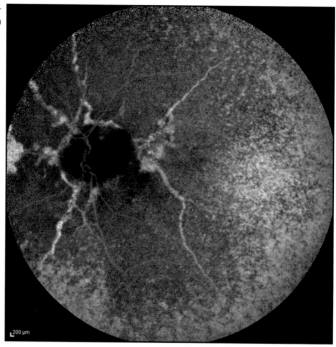

Figure 12-6. A patient presenting with a submacular hemorrhage underwent ICG imaging which showed a diffuse macular hypofluorescence from engorged choroidal vessels, but no focal hotspot to suggest the presence of a CNV.

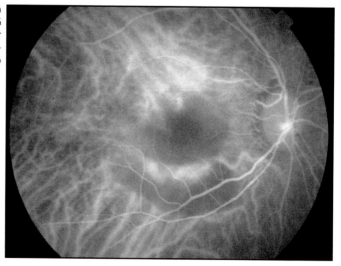

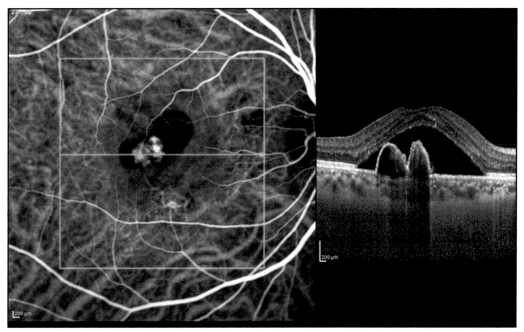

Figure 12-7. An ICG angiography image of the right eye of a 46-year-old man with polypoidal choroidal vasculopathy. Notice the hotspot with adjacent hemorrhage on the ICG image that corresponds to a pigment epithelial defect with surrounding subretinal fluid on optical coherence tomography.

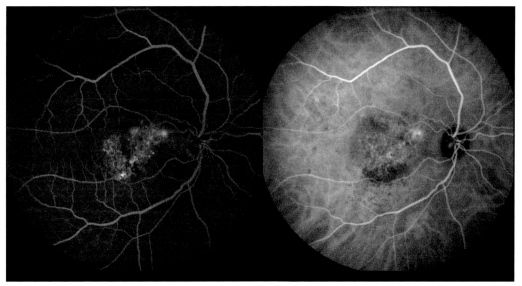

Figure 12-8. FA/ICG images showing a macular hotspot at the site of leakage in a patient with central serous retinopathy.

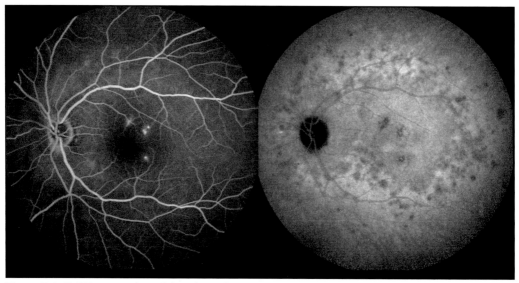

Figure 12-9. FA/ICG images of a syphilitic placoid lesion. There are areas of leakage in the FA which appear as hypo-fluorescent spots on the ICG.

13

FUNDUS AUTOFLUORESCENCE

Hasenin Al-khersan, MD
Ann Q. Tran, MD

Fundus autofluorescence (FAF) is an imaging technique for evaluating the integrity of the retinal pigment epithelium (RPE) based upon the condition of intrinsic intracellular fluorophores, lipofuscin granules. These fluorophores accumulate normally in functional RPE, but may be disturbed as a result of various pathologies.

Fluorescence occurs when a fluorophore absorbs a photon exciting an electron, which then releases a photon of longer wavelengths in order to return to its ground-state energy. When the fluorescent molecule is native to the tissue being illuminated, the term *autofluorescence* is applied. The emitted light is recorded, producing a brightness map showing the distribution of the fluorophores. Lipofuscin is the dominant macular fluorophore, occurring as a byproduct of the visual cycle with a peak excitation wavelength of 470 nanometers (nm) in the blue range. As the excited-state electron returns to ground-state, lipofuscin emits a photon of yellow-green light with a peak wavelength of 600 to 610 nm. Slightly longer wavelengths in the green range can be used to stimulate autofluorescence with small differences in the resulting images. Near-infrared autofluorescence which captures melanin-related fluorescence is stimulated by longer wavelengths in the range of 790 nm resulting in emissions in the range or 820 to 870 nm. These signals reveal more about the deeper structures in the choroid, are considerably weaker, and are used less commonly.

Fundus autofluorescence imaging can be performed on multiple imaging platforms:

- Fundus cameras
- Confocal scanning laser ophthalmoscopy (cSLO)
- Optos Ultra-Widefield cameras

Gologorsky D, Rosen RB, eds.
Principles of Ocular Imaging (pp 99-108).
© 2021 Taylor & Francis Group.

How to Interpret Fundus Autofluorescence

FAF images can exhibit areas of hyperfluorescence, hypofluorescence, or isofluorescence. Hyperfluorescence commonly results from abnormal lipofuscin accumulation within RPE cells due to decreased metabolism and turnover of photoreceptor byproducts. Hypofluorescence occurs secondary to decreased lipofuscin in RPE atrophy, as in geographic atrophy in age-related macular degeneration. Surrounding hypofluorescent lesions, perilesional hyperfluorescence often represents RPE dysfunction and can demonstrate variable patterns of hyperfluorescence.

Indications

- Age-related macular degeneration: drusen demonstrate variable effects on FAF depending on their size and effect on the surrounding RPE. Geographic atrophy in late stage age-related macular degeneration results in dense hypofluorescence representing RPE loss.

- Retinal and macular dystrophies: early vitelliform lesions of Best disease and macular flecks in Stargardt's disease are found to be highly autofluorescent. Early in the disease process, FAF may highlight findings not seen on clinical examination alone. Atrophy, which tends to occur in the later stages of these disease entities, presents with hypofluorescence.

- Plaquenil and hydroxychloroquine retinopathy: FAF can be particularly useful in tracking the progression of plaquenil toxicity. Initially, a perifoveal area of hyperfluorescence develops, representing photoreceptor death and accumulation of outer segments in the RPE. With progression, RPE death occurs, leading to confluent hypofluorescence.

- Optic disc drusen: FAF is useful in demonstrating the hyperfluorescence associated with optic disc drusen, which can be helpful in differentiating the condition from optic nerve edema and other pathologic entities.

- Choroidal melanoma: orange pigment overlying choroidal melanomas, representing intracellular lipofuscin, can be seen as hyperfluorescent on FAF. This pigment may not always be obvious on clinical exam and may be helpful in differentiating from a choroidal nevus.

- Central serous chorioretinopathy: subretinal fluid accumulation may initially present with increased autofluorescence in the acute stage as the RPE accumulates photoreceptor outer segments. With chronic disease, RPE cell loss may occur leading to a hypofluorescent pattern. The subretinal fluid may collect inferiorly in a gravity-dependent manner, a phenomenon termed "guttering."

- Inflammatory and infectious conditions: FAF is very useful in monitoring areas of activity. Conditions include syphilis, tuberculous, multiple evanescent white dot syndrome (MEWDS), serpiginous choroiditis, multifocal choroiditis, acute posterior multifocal placoid pigment epitheliopathy (APMPPE), etc.

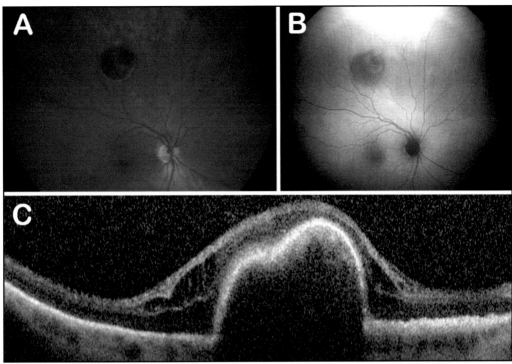

Figure 13-1. Hemorrhagic pigment epithelial detachment. (A) Fundus examination demonstrates a well-circumscribed, pigmented lesion with a yellow border representing a hemorrhagic pigment epithelial detachment. (B) FAF at the site of the detachment demonstrates hypofluorescence. (C) On optical coherence tomography (OCT), the pigment epithelial detachment can be seen with elevation and accompanying intraretinal fluid.

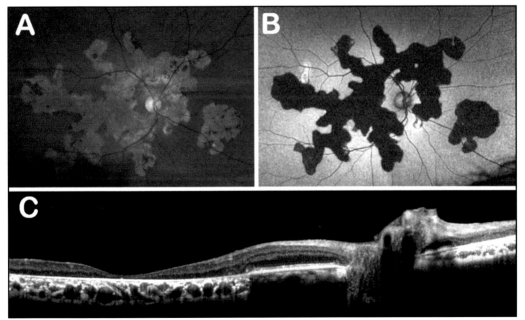

Figure 13-2. Serpiginous choroiditis. (A) Fundus examination demonstrates classic serpiginous lesions spreading centrifugally from the peripapillary area. (B) Active portions of the lesion, as seen inferonasal to the disc in this FAF, classically demonstrate a halo of hypofluorescence surrounding an area of hyperfluorescence. Inactive regions demonstrate starkly dark hypofluorescence with sharp margins. (C) OCT demonstrates corresponding retinal atrophy at the areas highlighted on the fundus photos and FAF.

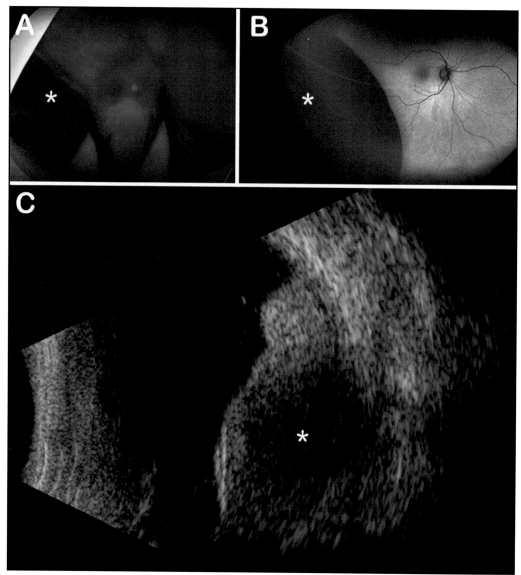

Figure 13-3. Uveal melanoma. (A) Funduscopic examination of the right eye demonstrates a large inferotemporal elevated pigmented lesion (asterisk). (B) FAF demonstrates stark hypofluorescence with elevations seen on (C) B-scan ultrasound.

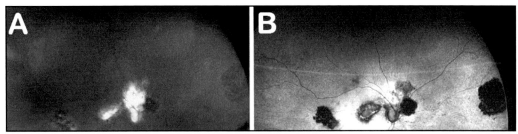

Figure 13-4. Tuberculosis chorioretinitis. (A) Fundus photo of inactive tuberculoid chorioretinal scarring. (B) FAF illustrates hypofluorescence scarring, and a hyperfluorescent lesion superior to the disc represents an area of active infection.

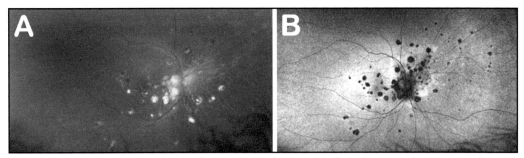

Figure 13-5. Multifocal choroiditis. (A) FAF demonstrates multiple punched-out chorioretinal scars. (B) FAF illustrates the corresponding hypofluorescent spots. Active lesions demonstrate hyperfluorescence before evolving into the pictured inactive hypofluorescent scars.

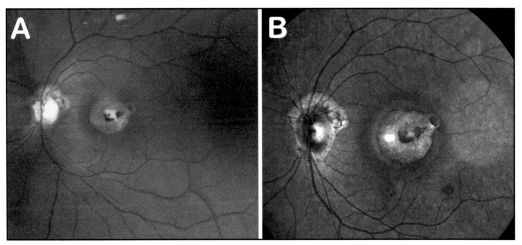

Figure 13-6. Best disease. (A) Fundus photo illustrates late-stage foveal atrophy with a central area of hyperpigmentation representing scarring from an old choroidal neovascular membrane. (B) FAF highlights foveal scarring as areas of dark hypofluorescence. The perifoveal area of retinal and RPE atrophy manifests as variable hyper- and hypofluorescence.

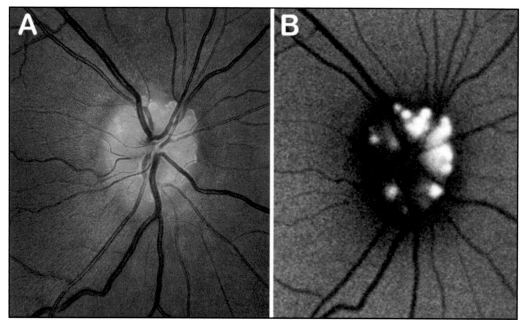

Figure 13-7. Optic disc drusen. (A) Fundus photo of optic disc drusen. (B) FAF highlights hyperfluorescent round or irregular structures within the optic nerve. The degree of fluorescence corresponds to the depth of these lesions within the optic nerve head, with buried drusen demonstrating less autofluorescence.

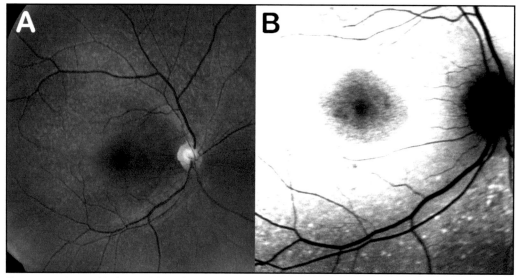

Figure 13-8. Stargardt's disease. (A) Fundus photo highlights characteristic flecks, seen here in the macula and mid-periphery. In the macula, there is darkening of the fovea. (B) FAF shows the flecks as areas of hyperfluorescence given the areas of lipofuscin accumulation in the RPE, while the areas of macular atrophy are hypofluorescent.

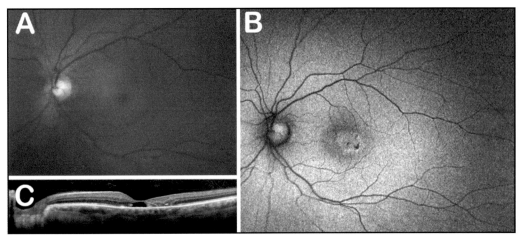

Figure 13-9. MacTel type 1. (A) Fundus photos show subtle areas of temporal hypopigmentation, more pronounced on (B) FAF as a surrounding ring of hypofluorescence corresponding to the loss of foveal luteal pigment. (C) OCT highlights the temporal loss of the outer nuclear layer and ellipsoid zone, causing an area of cavitation.

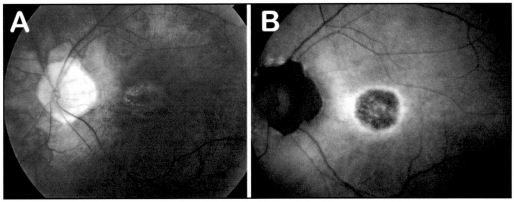

Figure 13-10. Bull's eye maculopathy. (A) Fundus photo shows advanced bull's eye maculopathy. (B) FAF shows a central area of hypopigmentation and surrounding hyperfluorescence corresponding to the RPE loss.

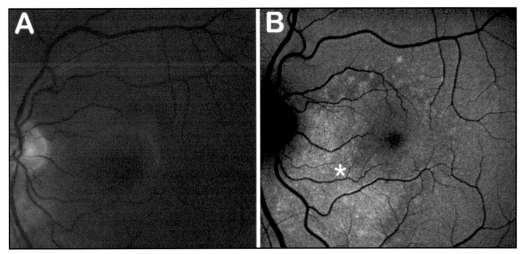

Figure 13-11. Neurosyphilis. (A) Fundus photo of a patient with subtle posterior placoid presentation of syphilis demonstrated more obviously on FAF (B) with areas of hyperfluorescence perifoveally (asterisk).

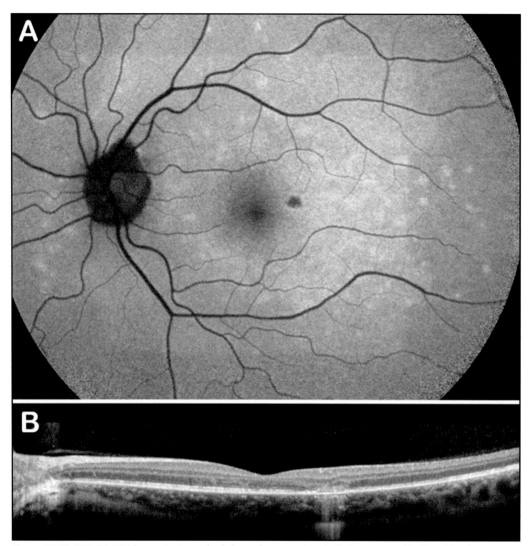

Figure 13-12. MEWDS. FAF demonstrates multiple hyperfluorescent spots that correspond to the white dots seen on clinical examination. On OCT, these lesions demonstrate granular disturbances in the region of ellipsoid zone or inner segment/outer segment junction. These characteristic hyperfluorescent dots may be more apparent on FAF than clinical examination in the early stage of onset, aiding in earlier diagnosis.

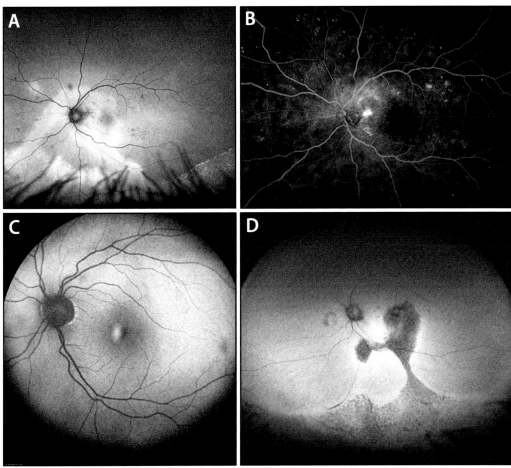

Figure 13-13. Central serous retinopathy (CSR). (A) FAF shows a hyperautofluorescent pattern inferiorly, secondary to the guttering from the accumulation of subretinal fluid. (B) Fluorescein angiography highlights a small focus of leakage temporally to the nerve. Alternative presentations of CSR include (C) variable central hyper- and hypofluorescence and (D) chronic CSR with hypofluorescence in a teardrop configuration.

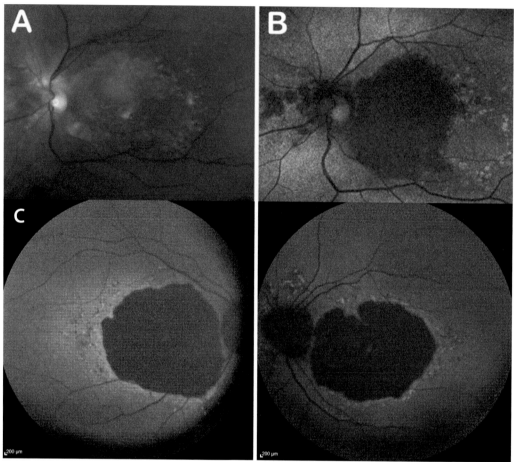

Figure 13-14. Dry age-related macular edema. (A) Fundus photo showing a large central area of geographic atrophy surrounded temporally by small yellow drusen. (B) On FAF, drusen may be hyperfluorescent, hypoflorescent, or isofluorescent, while areas of geographic atrophy are dark and hypofluorescent. (C) Another example of bilateral geographic atrophy on FAF.

14

OPTICAL COHERENCE TOMOGRAPHY IN RETINA

Daniel Gologorsky, MD, MBA

Optical coherence tomography (OCT) has become an increasingly invaluable imaging modality over the last two decades. It allows the clinician to obtain a cross-sectional view of the retina in high resolution, offering excellent detail of the vitreoretinal interface, retinal structures, retinal pigment epithelium, and choroid. In addition to a structural survey, recent advancements in OCT have allowed the clinician to perform quantitative volumetric and retinal thickness analyses to assist in diagnostics, disease progression assessments, and responses to therapy. In addition to the macula, OCT provides details of the optic nerve and anterior segment structures that provide critical imaging information for management of glaucoma and corneal diseases.

OCT is based upon the principle of low-coherence interferometry, which measures the backscattering of light directed into biological tissues to reconstruct high-resolution, cross-sectional images of the illuminated tissue. Information on the intensity and the delay of reflected light is useful for characterizing the tissue being imaged. The illuminating light source of the OCT is an infrared scanning beam that passes through a beam splitter on its way to the subject of interest. The light is divided into a reference arm and a sample arm. Once it reflects from the tissue, light returning to the sample arm is reunited with the light from the reference arm, resulting in various degrees of interference which changes the signal amplitude. These different sequential longitudinal signals are called *A-scans*, and composites of these scans can be assembled into a transverse cross-sectional image, or a *B-scan*.

Backscattered light can be detected in a time-domain (TD) arrangement, which uses a moveable reference target within the interferometer, or with a Fourier-domain (FD) arrangement with a fixed reference arm. With a FD arrangement the variation in the light returning can be measured with a spectrometer, so-called spectral-domain (SD) OCT, or the light source itself may sweep through a range of frequencies, so-called swept-source (SS) OCT. In FD

Gologorsky D, Rosen RB, eds.
Principles of Ocular Imaging (pp 109-117).
© 2021 Taylor & Francis Group.

devices, the simultaneous collection of data translates to a dramatic increase in scanning speed, allowing for greater data acquisition and fewer motion artifacts. TD-OCT devices perform 400 A-scans/second, while spectral domain devices can produce 18,000 to 100,000 A-scans/second. Moreover, this faster speed of data acquisition allows the OCT to cover a larger 6 × 6 mm of retina, sufficiently dense to capture a three-dimensional cube of tissue. SD-OCT typically utilizes a wider bandwidth light source than TD-OCT, which allows for increased axial resolving power -5 μm (down to 2 μm) for SD-OCT, while TD-OCT usually resolves up to 10 microns. SS-OCT is faster than SD-OCT (100,000 to 3,000,000 scans/second) and utilizes longer wavelengths, allowing for deeper tissue penetration for applications such as enhanced choroidal or vitreous imaging, but at the expense of lower-axial resolution than SD-OCT. Currently, SS-OCT is more expensive but is steadily gaining market share as of this time.

OCT can be very helpful for evaluating the health of the choroid. Choroidal thickness varies in a number of pathologies and provides valuable diagnostic information. For example, patients with central serous retinopathy or polypoidal choroidal vasculopathy have been described to have a thickened choroid (pachychoroid), while patients with macular degeneration, myopic degeneration, or retinitis pigmentosa typically have an attenuated choroid. Enhanced depth imaging OCT (EDI-OCT) is an imaging technique that expanded the apparent depth of field by moving the point of focus deeper into the retinal tissue, which enhances the signal from the deeper choroidal structures. The EDI arrangement re-inverts an inverted portion of the image to extend the limited depth of focus of SD-OCT. This improved visualization of the choroid and choroidal-scleral junction allows improved measurement of choroidal thickness.

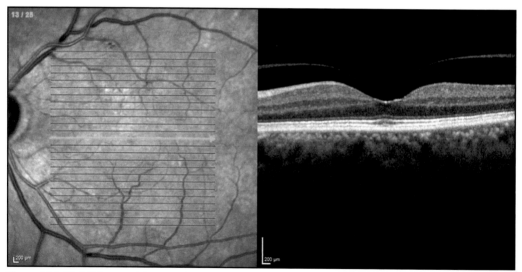

Figure 14-1. SD-OCT image of the normal retina. The retinal layers, photoreceptors, retinal pigment epithelium (RPE), and choroid are distinct and undisrupted by edema, hemorrhage, or neovascular membranes. The vitreous face is partially detached from the surface of the macula, adhering only to a small area within the foveal depression.

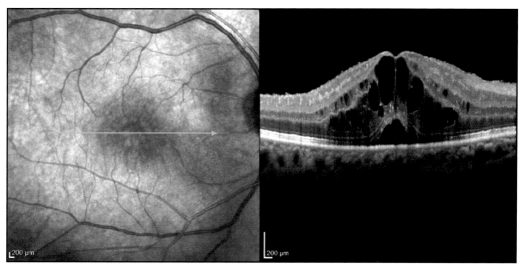

Figure 14-2. Cystoid macular edema in a patient following cataract surgery. Note the petaloid pattern of fluid accumulation within the outer plexiform layer.

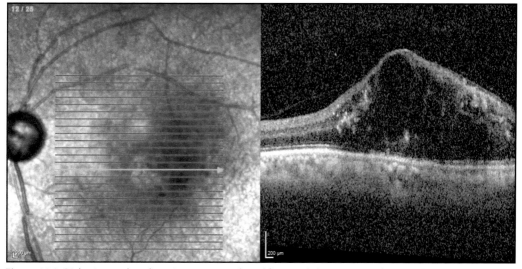

Figure 14-3. Diabetic macular edema in a patient with proliferative diabetic retinopathy. Note the signal attenuation due to vitreous hemorrhage and debris.

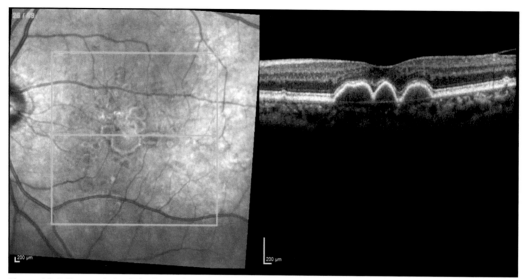

Figure 14-4. Nonexudative ("dry") macular degeneration with drusen. Note the thin choroid.

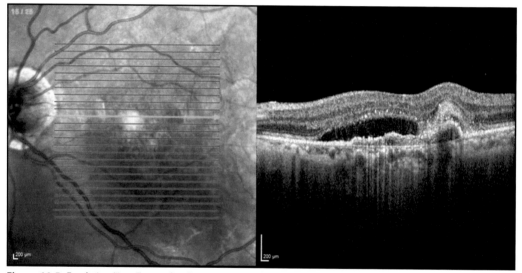

Figure 14-5. Exudative ("wet") macular degeneration with hemorrhage, edema, and choroidal neovascular membranes.

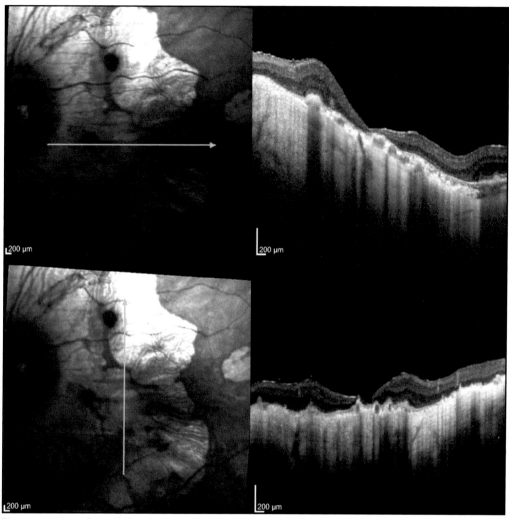

Figure 14-6. OCT of a staphylomatous eye with extensive RPE atrophy and loss of outer segments. Note the myopic macular hole.

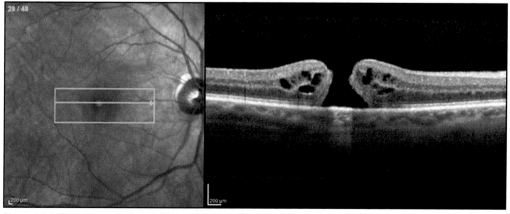

Figure 14-7. Stage 4 macular hole with hyaloid separation, cystoid hydration, full-thickness rupture, and RPE lucency.

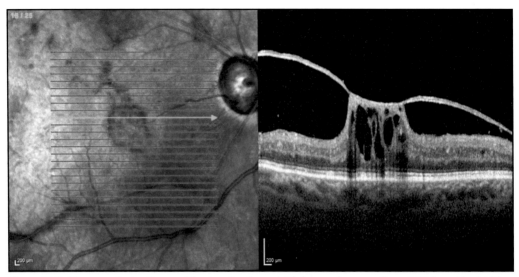

Figure 14-8. Vitreomacular traction resulting in extensive cystoid changes from an adherent thickened hyaloid face in a patient with 20/25 vision.

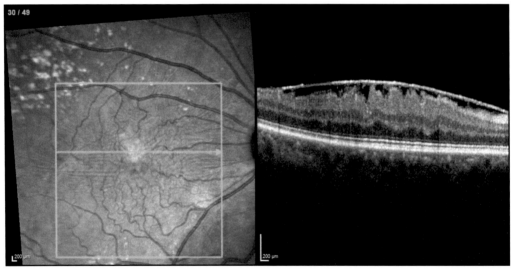

Figure 14-9. A taut epiretinal membrane puckering the macular surface in a patient with prior surgery for retinal detachment repair.

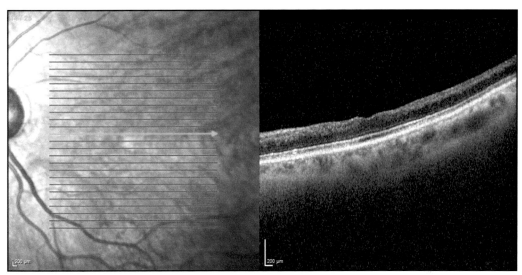

Figure 14-10. OCT revealing severely attenuated inner retinal layers several months after a central retinal artery occlusion.

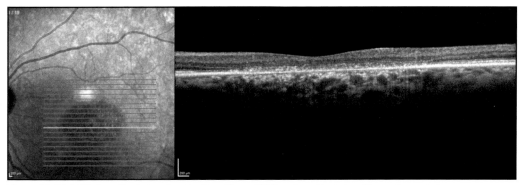

Figure 14-11. OCT of a patient showing significant loss of RPE and resultant signal hyper-transmission.

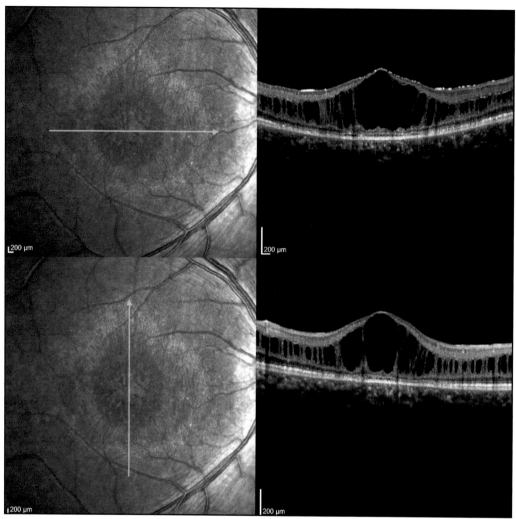

Figure 14-12. OCT of X-linked retinoschisis showing schisis cavities through various layers of the macula. Typical radial pattern is seen in the infrared fundus image.

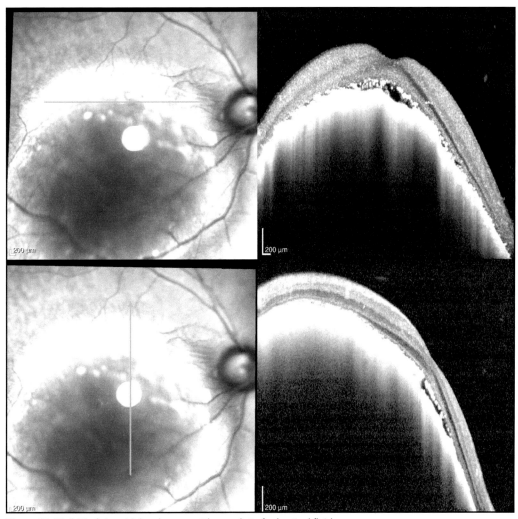

Figure 14-13. OCT of choroidal melanoma with a pocket of subretinal fluid.

15

Optical Coherence Tomography Angiography

Chris Y. Wu, MD
Richard B. Rosen, MD

Optical coherence tomography (OCT), first reported in 1991, has become indispensable for retinal imaging and clinical management of retinal disease. Yielding in vivo cross-sectional images with near-histological resolution, OCT can non-invasively reveal the subtlest quantitative features of macular and optic nerve head anatomy. OCT utilizes interference patterns of infrared light reconstructed to generate cross-sectional images of the retina in a variety of perspectives, analogous to the way ultrasonic images are generated.

Optical coherence tomography angiography (OCTA) is a functional imaging modality, derived from recently available forms of high speed OCT, that employs small differences between sequential scans to reconstruct the motion of blood flow. Images rendered in the en face perspective reveal angiographic maps of capillary blood flow based upon this "motion contrast" as opposed to the contrast studies using exogenous dyes such as fluorescein or indocyanine green. Motion contrast can be derived using different algorithms (eg, split-spectrum amplitude decorrelation angiography, speckle variance, phase variance) to improve the signal-to-noise ratio and minimize artifacts from other sources of movement. The resulting images can isolate layers of the retina using image segmentation to display blood vessel plexi from different layers of the retina independently. This is in contrast to fluorescein angiography, which displays the larger vessels along with the superficial capillary plexus. The high resolution and consistent quality of the images enables quantification of various perfusion metrics from the en face images, such as vessel density, flow index, and foveal avascular zone size. Current commercial OCTA systems have an optical axial resolution of 5 to 10 μm and transverse resolution of ~20 μm.

Axial segmentation of the macula is typically divided into four en face zones of OCTA, the superficial capillary plexus (capillary network of the ganglion cell layer and nerve fiber layer), the deep capillary plexus (capillary network situated between the outer boundary of the inner plexi-

Gologorsky D, Rosen RB, eds.
Principles of Ocular Imaging (pp 119-134).
© 2021 Taylor & Francis Group.

form layer and the midpoint of the outer plexiform layer with section thickness of 55 μm), the outer retina (photoreceptors, usually avascular), and the choriocapillaris (capillary network situated in a 30 μm section immediately beneath the retinal pigment epithelium). Some OCTA systems also offer segmentation boundaries which isolate the intermediate capillary plexus between the superficial and deep capillary layers. The ability to isolate these physiologic networks uniquely enables the recognition and imaging of neovascular membranes at different levels, much better than with any exogenous contrast angiography. OCTA is also uniquely capable of imaging the radial peripapillary capillary network within the retinal nerve fiber layer extending from the optic disc. This feature offers a sensitive means of characterizing glaucomatous damage especially in the very early and very advanced stages. Automated segmentation, while not standardized between various commercial OCTA systems, provides default boundaries that may require manual adjustments to compensate for pathological disturbances. Image areas range from 2 × 2 mm to 12 × 12 m with currently available OCTA devices.

OCTA has only recently become available and has certain limitations in its current form. Instead of showing various forms of leakage, as seen in exogenous dye angiograms, it reveals the fine structure of any abnormal vessels present. Other challenges stem from the speed of the current systems, which limit the exam to subjects with steady fixation and relatively central pathology. Projection and movement artifacts, inability to see vessels with slow vascular flow below detection threshold, limited depth of penetration, and smaller immediate field of view are also issues which have slowed clinical incorporation. Interpretation of the clinical significance of previously unrecognized pathology (eg, early nonexudative subclinical neovascular lesions in dry age-related macular degeneration, retinal and choroidal flow voids) are current issues of controversy. As the hardware and software of OCTA continues to evolve, it promises to improve our care of our patients due to its rapidity, noninvasive nature, low cost, and depth-resolving access to the finest capillary networks of the eye.

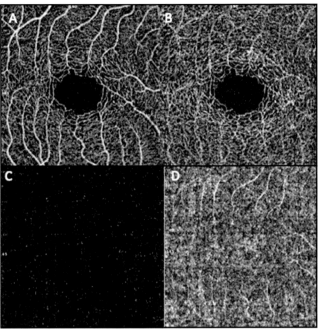

Figure 15-1. (A) Superficial capillary plexus, (B) deep capillary plexus, (C) outer retina, (D) and choriocapillaris from OCTA scan (Angiovue, Optovue) of normal patient. Note the absence of blood vessels in the outer retina C. Projection artifact from large superficial vessels are noted in the deep capillary plexus and choriocapillaris.

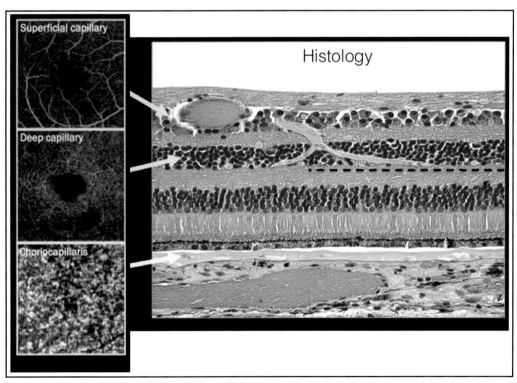

Figure 15-2. Segmented retinal vascular layers from OCTA correlated with cross-sectional histological image. (Reprinted with permission from Agemy SA, Scripsema NK, Shah CM, et al, 2015.)

Figure 15-3. Superficial capillary plexus of patient with diabetic retinopathy. OCTA reveals all vasculopathic details of diabetic retinopathy. See: microaneurysms (red arrows); vascular loops (blue arrow); nonperfusion (green arrow); FAZ erosion (white arrow); venous beading (yellow arrow); neovascularization (orange arrow); multiple capillary beds (pink arrow).

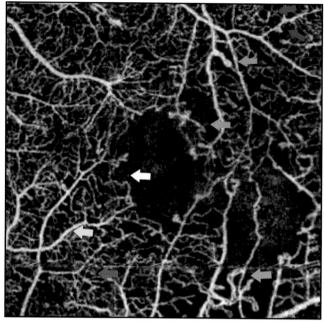

Figure 15-4. Foveal superficial OCTA images from control, patient with diabetes without retinopathy, nonproliferative, and proliferative diabetic retinopathy patients. With increasing stage of diabetic retinopathy, note the increased microvascular abnormalities on OCTA; specifically, there is an enlarging acircular foveal avascular zone, a capillary nonperfusion, and microaneurysms.

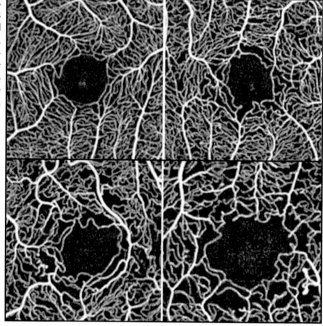

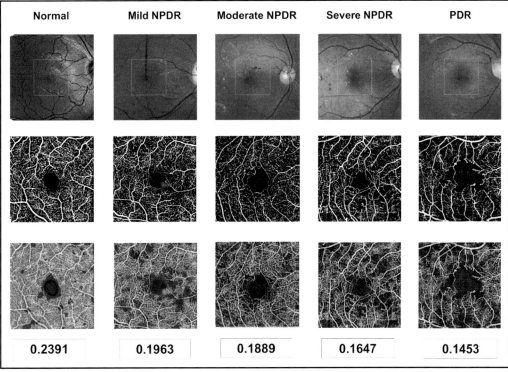

Figure 15-5. A series of fundus photos, superficial capillary angiograms, and color-coded vascular perfusion maps (blue represents absence of perfusion) from control and diabetic retinopathy patients. Qualitative and quantitative changes in the fundus photos, angiograms, and perfusion maps are noted as the images progress from normal eyes to proliferative diabetic retinopathy patients. Bottom numbers show perfusion indices. (Reprinted with permission from Agemy SA, Scripsema NK, Shah CM, et al, 2015.)

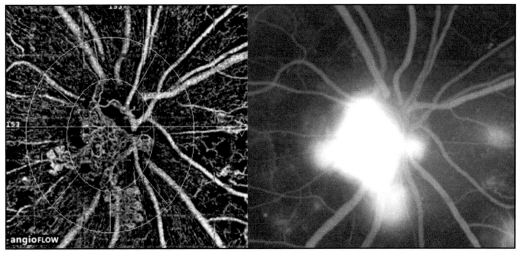

Figure 15-6. Peripapillary OCTA showing optic disc neovascularization in proliferative diabetic retinopathy patient. Corresponding fluorescein angiography shows image degradation due to leaking fluorescein dye.

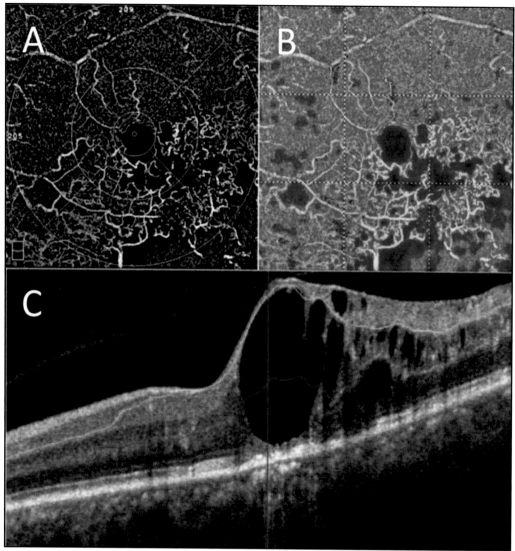

Figure 15-7. OCTA and spectral-domain OCT from patient with branch retinal vein occlusion complicated by cystoid macular edema. (A) OCTA image shows capillary remodelling and capillary nonperfusion, which corresponds to (B) dark blue areas on color-coded perfusion map. (C) OCT shows retinal thickening and cystoid macular edema.

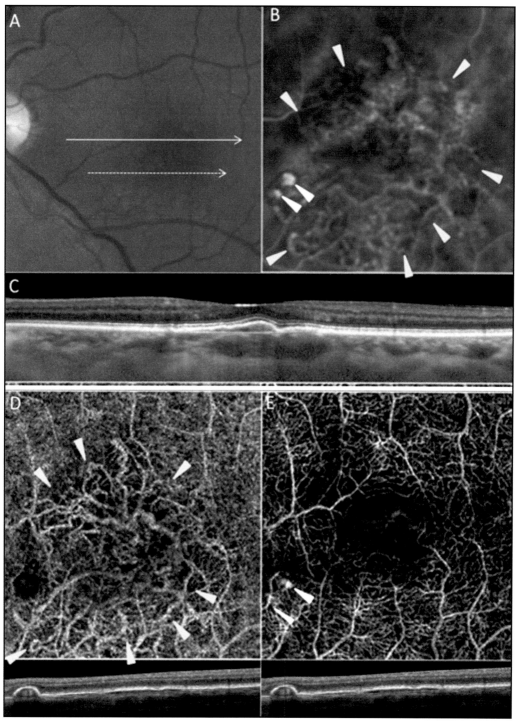

Figure 15-8. (A) Color fundus photo, (B) indocyanine green (ICG) angiography, (C) OCT, and (D) OCTA segmented to show choriocapillaris and (E) deep capillary plexus from patient with polypoidal choroidal vasculopathy. Note the branching vascular network colored red and outlined by yellow arrowheads on ICG (B) and OCTA (D). Polyps are denoted by white arrowheads (B). OCT (C) shows fibrovascular pigment epithelial detachment with underlying large choroidal pachyvessel. (Reprinted with permission from Maiko Inoue, Chandrakumar Balaratnasingam, and K. Bailey Freund.)

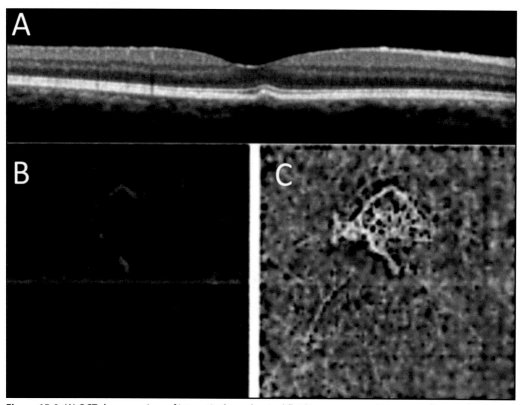

Figure 15-9. (A) OCT shows no signs of intraretinal or subretinal fluid in asymptomatic patient with drusen. (B) OCTA segmented to outer retina and (C) choriocapillaris shows type 1 choroidal neovascularization (CNV) in the choriocap-illaris. Treatment of nonexudative asymptomatic neovascular lesions in dry age-related macular degeneration is still controversial. (Reprinted with permission from Nehemy MB, Brocchi DN, Veloso CE, 2015.)

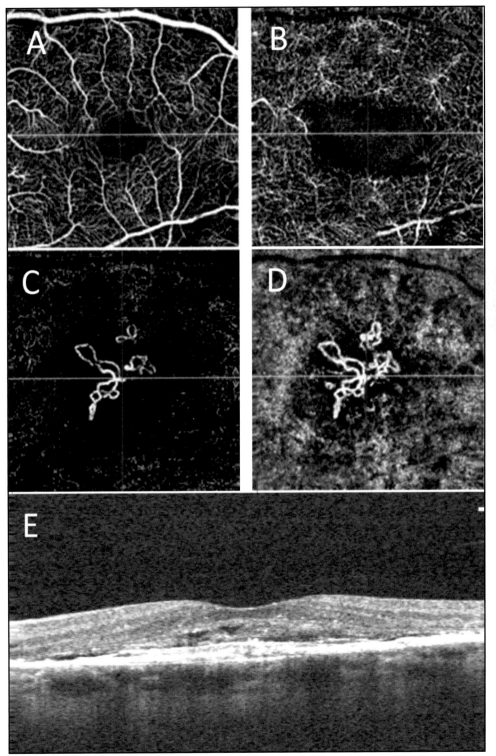

Figure 15-10. OCTA demonstrating type 2 subretinal CNV. (A) OCTA of the superficial capillary plexus, (B) deep capillary plexus, (C) outer retina, and (D) choriocapillaris. Lacy neovascular network is seen in (C) normally avascular retina and (D) in the choriocapillaris. (E) Structural OCT shows subretinal hyperreflective plaque. (Reprinted with permission from Bruno Lumbroso.)

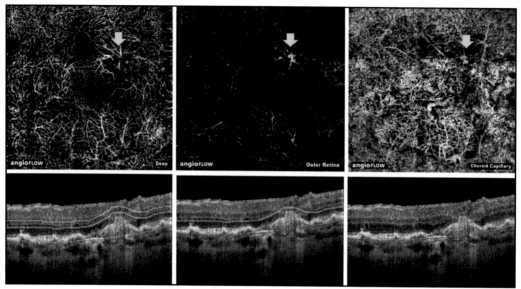

Figure 15-11. OCTA images shows type 3 CNV (retinal angiomatous proliferation). Intraretinal and inner choroidal components of lesion are highlighted in red and denoted by blue arrow.

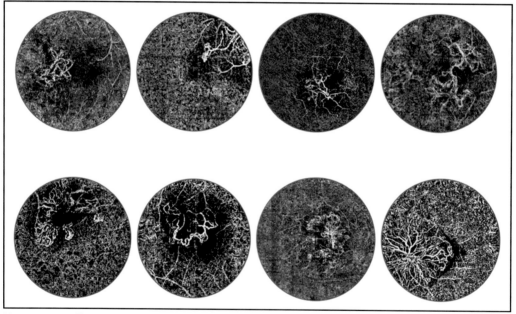

Figure 15-12. Different branching patterns of CNV on OCTA. (Reprinted with permission from André Romano.)

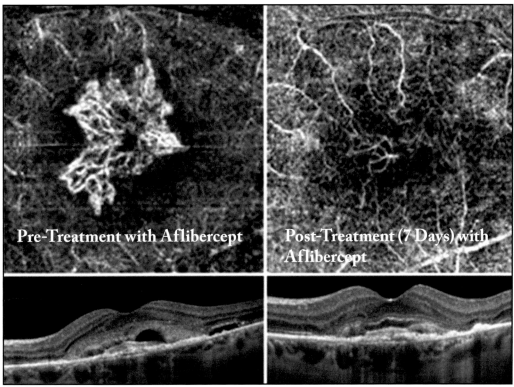

Figure 15-13. OCTA and OCT shows regression of CNV and subretinal fluid after treatment with aflibercept. (Reprinted with permission from Bruno Lumbroso.)

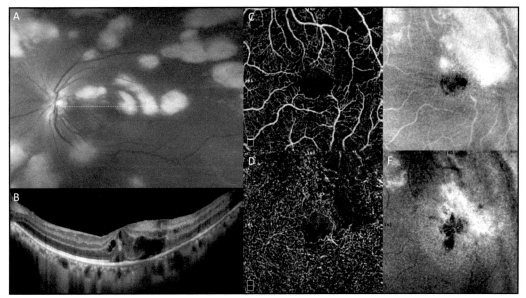

Figure 15-14. (A) Widefield photo from patient with progressive outer retinal necrosis showing multifocal outer retinal opacification and scattered intraretinal hemorrhages. (B) OCT shows thickening, cystoid changes, and areas inner retinal hyperreflectivity corresponding to progressive outer retinal necrosis lesions. (C, D) OCTA and en face OCT shows perifoveal capillary nonperfusion (E, F) corresponding to hyperreflective areas on en face OCT. (Reprinted with permission from Wu CY, Garcia P, Rosen RB, 2019.)

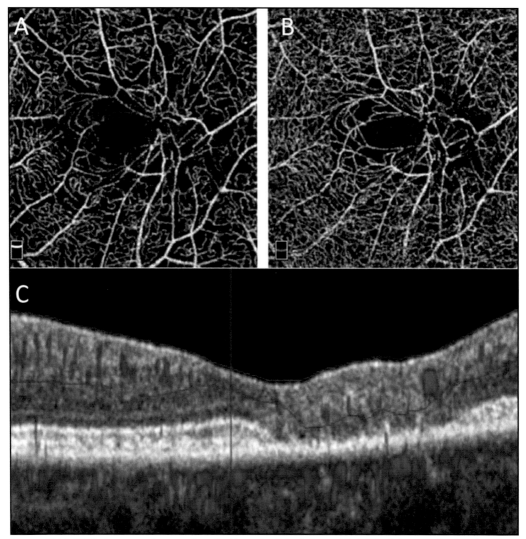

Figure 15-15. OCTA demonstrating macular telangiectasia of the left eye. (A) OCTA of the superficial and (B) deep capillary plexus with (C) cross-sectional structural OCT with angioflow. Note the juxtafoveal areas of capillary nonperfusion in the superficial and deep capillary plexus (especially temporal juxtafoveal area), corresponding to atrophic changes on OCT. (OCTA Gallery, slide 4.)

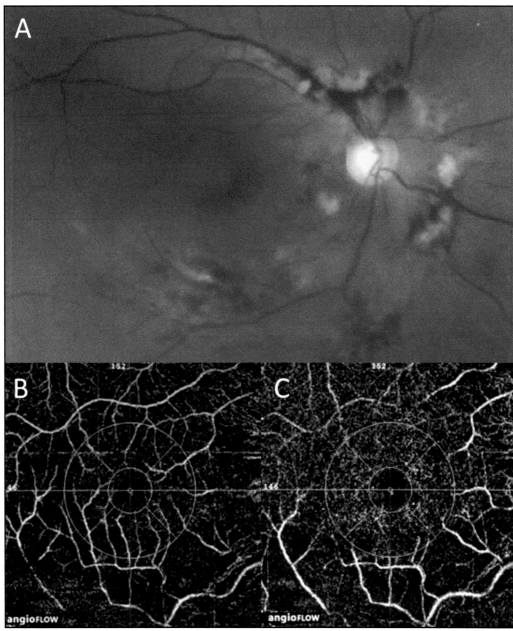

Figure 15-16. Images from patient with cytomegalovirus retinitis. (A) Fundus photo shows intraretinal hemorrhages and fluffy retinitis lesions. (B) OCTA shows confluent areas of capillary nonperfusion in superficial and (C) deep capillary plexus.

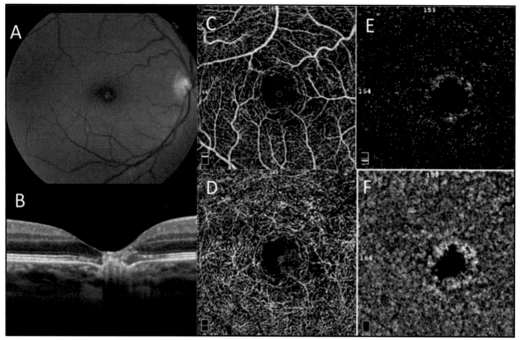

Figure 15-17. Laser injury from patient who accidentally looked into the exit aperture of a repetitively pulsed infrared Nd:YAG 1064 nanometer laser. (A) Fundus photo shows foveal atrophic scar. (B) OCT shows central replacement of photoreceptor structures with hyperreflective scarring. (C) OCTA of superficial and (D) deep capillary plexus shows juxtafoveal capillary nonperfusion. (F) OCTA of choriocapillaris shows central circular area of nonperfusion.

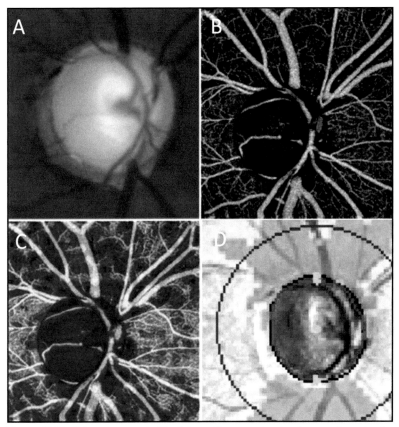

Figure 15-18. Color photograph (A) of the optic nerve showing increased cup-to-disc ratio consistent with glaucoma. (B) Peripapillary OCTA and (C) color-coded perfusion map shows peripapillary capillary nonperfusion and perfusion deficits (dark blue), respectively. (D) Peripapillary OCT shows retinal nerve fiber layer thinning in areas of decreased perfusion.

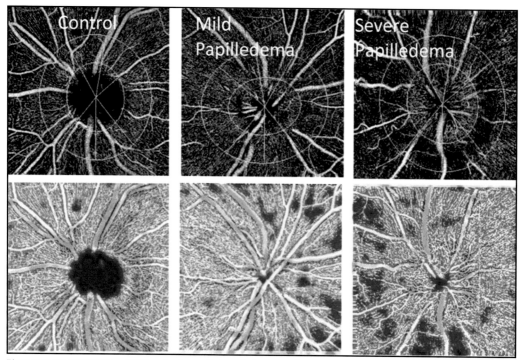

Figure 15-19. Peripapillary OCTA and color-coded perfusion map shows worsening perfusion deficits (in dark blue) as severity of papilledema increases.

16

ADAPTIVE OPTICS

Chris Y. Wu, MD
Richard B. Rosen, MD

Adaptive optics (AO) is a technology for correcting wavefront distortions that reduce the resolution of an image. It was originally developed for ground-based astronomical telescopes "to remove the twinkle from the stars." When added to the ophthalmoscope, it can acquire in vivo images of cellular structures in the human eye with an optical lateral resolution of 2 μm or less. Images with this resolution were previously only obtainable on histological specimens. Early attempts at AO imaging in the 1980s and 1990s at the University of Heidelberg using a scanning light ophthalmoscope (SLO), invented in 1980, showed that a deformable mirror could change the shape of its surface to compensate for optical distortions of the eye and enhance the resolution of retinal imaging devices. Imaging quality was subsequently improved when researchers incorporated a Shack-Hartmann wavefront sensor with a deformable mirror in the optical path of an SLO. This advance enabled compensation for higher-order wavefront aberrations, in addition to lower-order aberrations such as defocus and astigmatism.

The first in vivo imaging of human cone photoreceptors was achieved in 1997 using an AO-fundus camera. Currently, AO systems utilize a wavefront sensor coupled to a wavefront shaping device, usually a deformable mirror, that can modify the wavefront of the beam of imaging light using software. AO systems have been combined with a variety of optical systems, including fundus cameras (employing flood illumination), scanning light ophthalmoscopes (employing either a flying spot or line scanner), and optical coherence tomography (OCT). The adaptive optics scanning light ophthalmoscope (AOSLO) offers increased contrast relative to the AO-fundus camera, which allows the detection of both singly and multiply scattered light, and can employ a variety of contrast agents (eg, single photon and multiphoton fluorescence, extrinsic dye-based or intrinsic motion contrast). The resolution of AOSLOs have now reached the diffraction limit for normal

Gologorsky D, Rosen RB, eds.
Principles of Ocular Imaging (pp 135-147).
© 2021 Taylor & Francis Group.

eyes with clear optical media. Detection schemes for AOSLO include confocal and non-confocal (eg, large pinhole, offset pinhole, dark-field, split-detector) methods.

In vivo images acquired using AO have enhanced our visualization and understanding of photoreceptors (both cones and rods), retinal vasculature, retinal ganglion cells and nerve fiber layer, retinal pigment epithelium, mural cells, glial and other retinal cells, and the lamina cribrosa. While adoption of AO has been generally limited to research labs and clinical research settings, continued development of AO technology holds promise of overcoming the many current limitations that hinder its widespread adoption into clinical practice. Currently, these limitations include extended time of acquisition, post-processing demands, system expense, limited field of view, and optical restrictions related to media opacities, such as cataract, high refractive errors, unstable fixation, poor tear film quality, and pseudophakia.

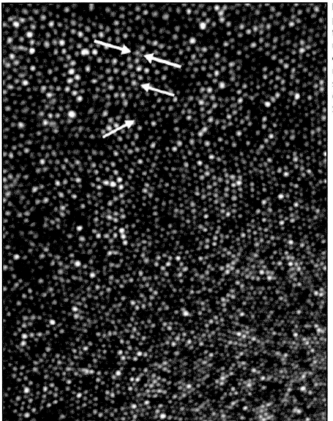

Figure 16-1. Normal images of human photoreceptor mosaic collected with confocal AOSLO. The arrows point to some rod photoreceptors closest to the foveal center, which is located at the bottom right center. The rods are significantly smaller than the cone photoreceptors. (Reprinted with permission from Dubra A, Sulai Y, Norris JL, et al., 2011.)

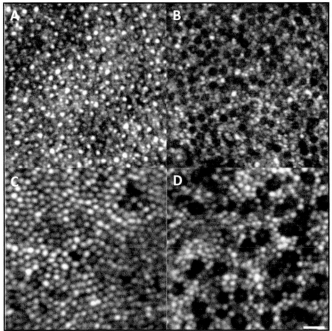

Figure 16-2. AOSLO images of photoreceptor mosaic in (A) healthy patient, (B) sildenafil toxic maculopathy, (C) retinitis pigmentosa, and (D) cone-rod dystrophy. Dark non-waveguiding cone and rod photoreceptors are seen in B through D.

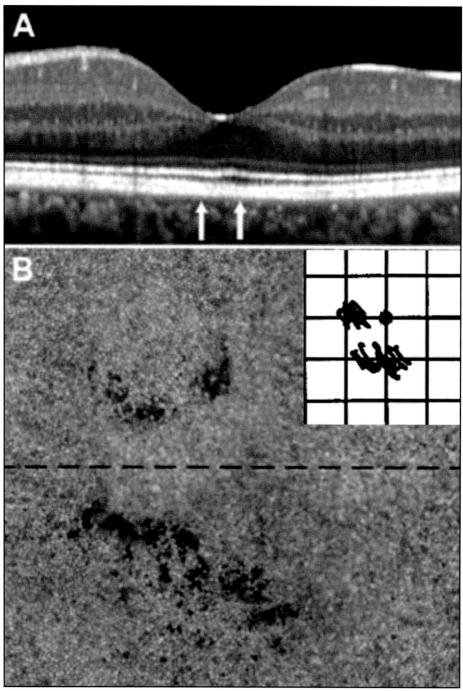

Figure 16-3. AOSLO montage images showing photoreceptor mosaic defects following closed globe blunt trauma. The patient had visual complaints despite normal clinical imaging with OCT. (A) The two areas of photoreceptor disruption corresponded to the patient's subjective flickering scotomas on Amsler grid. (B) The flickering was due to the site of the injury being in the dominant eye, which incited retinal rivalry with the unaffected better-seeing, but nondominant, eye. Dashed black lines indicate the location of corresponding OCT. (Reprinted with permission from Flatter JA, Cooper RF, Dubow MJ, et al., 2014.)

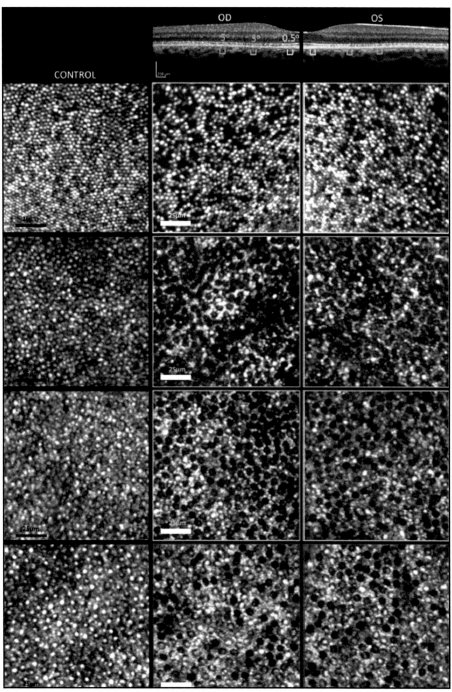

Figure 16-4. Images from a young patient who presented with bilateral multicolored photopsias and erythropsia (red-tinted vision) after taking a toxic dose of off-label sildenafil citrate purchased from the Internet. OCT of both eyes shows irregularities of the ellipsoid zone associated with thinning and poor delineation of the interdigitation zone. AOSLO images show multiple dark spots in the cone mosaic corresponding to non-waveguiding cones at increasing eccentricities from the foveal center in both eyes. (Reprinted with permission from Yanoga F, Gentile RC, Chui TYP, et al., 2018.)

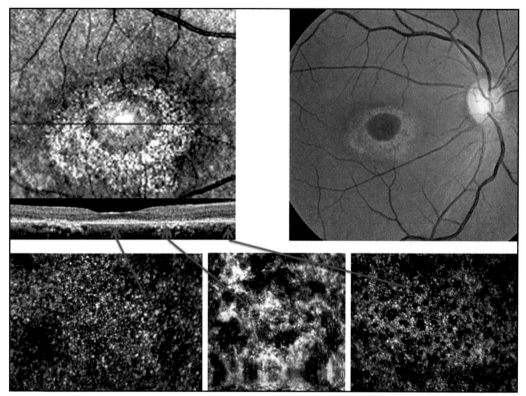

Figure 16-5. Chloroquine maculopathy: standard fundus photo, en face OCT, and AOSLO. The fundus photo and en face OCT images (top row) show a classic bull's eye pattern of perifoveal atrophy. The AOSLO images (bottom row) from different regions in the area of atrophy show disruption of photoreceptor mosaic.

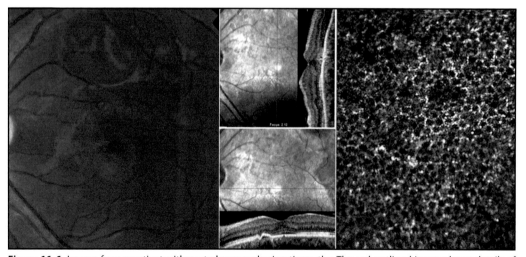

Figure 16-6. Images from a patient with central serous chorioretinopathy. The red-outlined image shows details of the retinal pigment epithelium (RPE) mosaic, normally obscured in AO due to the high reflectance of the photoreceptors. The small amount of subretinal fluid lifting the photoreceptors allows clear delineation of the RPE cell borders.

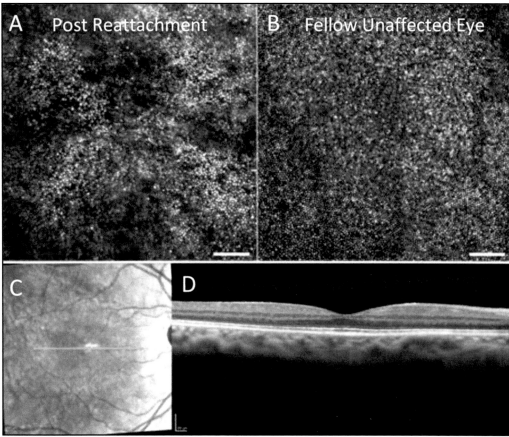

Figure 16-7. (A, B) AOSLO, (C) infrared, and (D) OCT images taken from patient who had a macula-involving retinal detachment surgically repaired. Although there was no subretinal fluid and the OCT images appeared normal, dark patches of non-waveguiding photoreceptors are noted on the AOSLO image A. The measured cone density on AOSLO images corresponds to best-corrected visual acuity after macula-off retinal detachment repair.

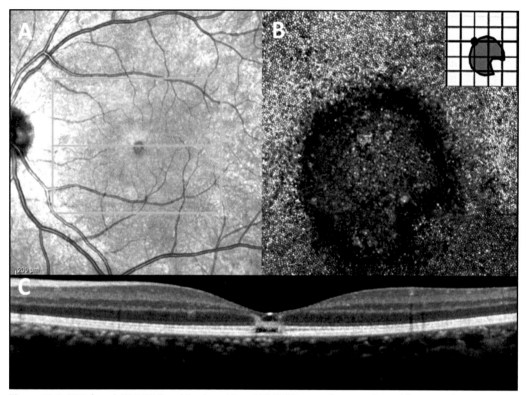

Figure 16-8. (A) Infrared, (B) AOSLO and Amsler grid, and (C) OCT images from a patient with acute solar retinopathy. The infrared (A) photo shows a central area of hyporeflectivity. The OCT C image shows near full-thickness hyperreflectivity at the foveal center with hyporeflectivity of inner and outer segments. The AOSLO image B shows an area of dark non-waveguiding photoreceptors that corresponds in shape to a partial solar eclipse and to the patient's scotoma (flipped vertically) on the Amsler grid. (Reprinted with permission from Wu CY, Jansen ME, Andrade J, et al, 2018.)

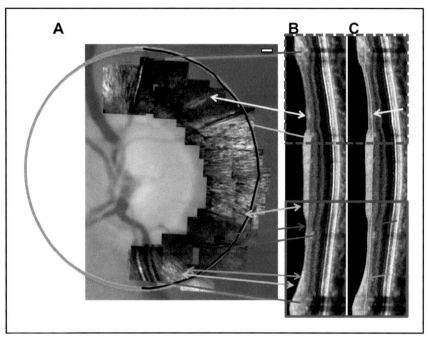

Figure 16-9. Montage of peripapillary AOSLO images superimposed upon the fundus photograph. (A) The green circle indicates the location of the OCT circumpapillary scans, and the black semicircle indicates the temporal half of this scan. (B) The temporal portion of the OCT circumpapillary scan is shown without and (C) with the retinal nerve fiber layer bundles marked. The purple lines extending to (A) indicate corresponding blood vessels. (Reprinted with permission from Hood DC, Chen MF, Lee D, et al., 2015.)

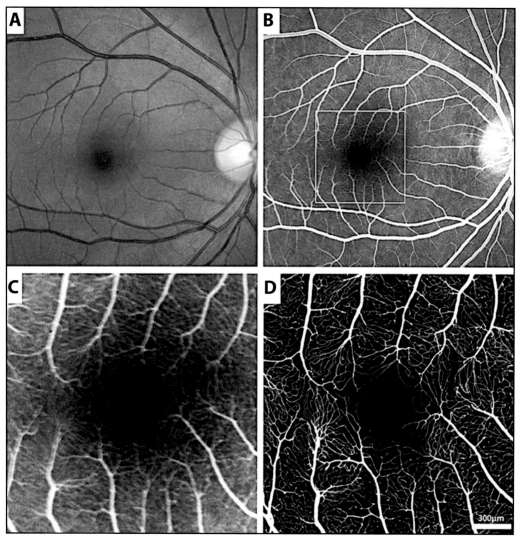

Figure 16-10. (A) Standard color fundus photo, (B) standard field fluorescein angiography (FA), (C) magnified conventional FA, and (D) magnified AOSLO FA from normal patient demonstrating the significant resolution enhancement produced by the addition of adaptive optics.

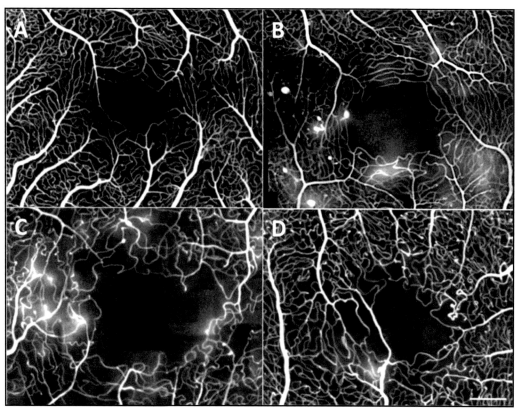

Figure 16-11. Magnified AOSLO FA of (A) normal patient, (B) diabetic retinopathy, (C) central retinal vein occlusion, and (D) sickle cell retinopathy. The pathologic images (B through D) are remarkable for capillary nonperfusion, microaneurysms, enlarged foveal avascular zone, and leakage of dye.

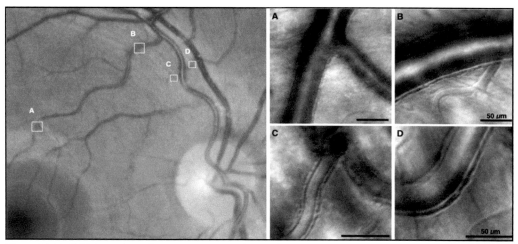

Figure 16-12. (A-D) Arteriolar wall structures in normal control patient on a color fundus photo and AOSLO.

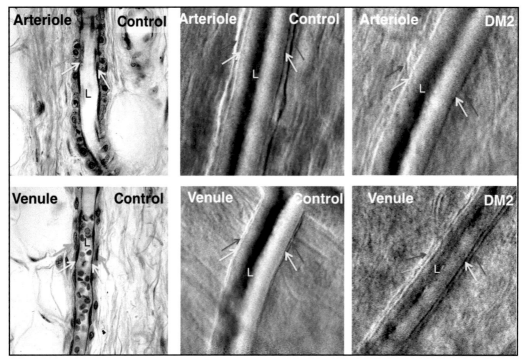

Figure 16-13. Histologic and AOSLO images from control patients and a patient with type 2 diabetes mellitus, demonstrating the arteriolar and venular wall thickening in the patient with diabetes as compared to control patients.

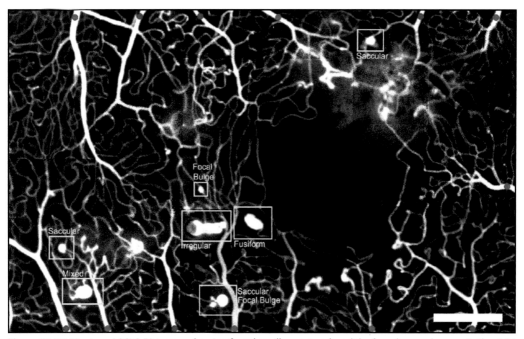

Figure 16-14. Montage AOSLO FA images showing foveal capillary network and the foveal avascular zone in the right eye of a patient with hypertension. Microaneurysms of various size and morphology are visible. Red dots indicate arterioles. Blue dots indicate venules. Scale bar: 300 µm.

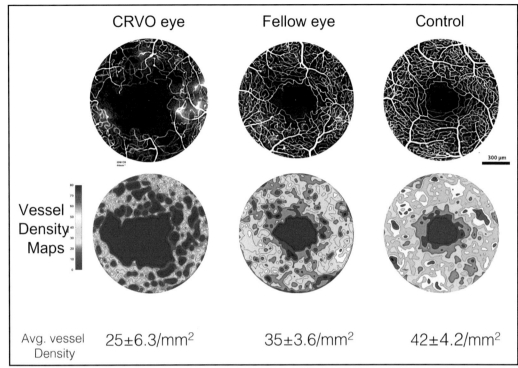

CRVO eye	Fellow eye	Control

Vessel Density Maps

Avg. vessel Density	$25\pm6.3/mm^2$	$35\pm3.6/mm^2$	$42\pm4.2/mm^2$

Figure 16-15. AOSLO FA and vessel density maps from the affected eye and fellow eye of a patient with central retinal vein occlusion compared to a normal control subject. AOSLO FA image from eye with central retinal vein occlusion shows capillary nonperfusion, leakage, enlarged foveal avascular zone, and telangiectatic capillaries with corresponding perfusion deficits on density map. Fellow eye also demonstrates significant perfusion deficits in the asymptomatic eye compared to vessel density map of normal patient's eye. (Reprinted with permission from Pinhas A, Dubow M, Shah N, et al, 2015.)

17

Microperimetry

Hasenin Al-khersan, MD
Thomas Lazzarini, MD
Ann Q. Tran, MD

Microperimetry, also known as fundus-related perimetry, is a visual field test that maps retinal sensitivity at designated points on the retina. Similar to standard automated perimetry used in glaucoma testing, this test presents light stimuli of various luminance levels to a grid of points on the retina, creating a map of stimulus sensitivity of the fundus. The test relies on the patient's ability to respond and indicate recognition of a stimulus, which can limit the reliability of the test. Concurrently, the test tracks and captures real-time images of the fundus using either scanning laser or fundus photography. The resultant retinal sensitivity map is overlaid onto fundus image.

Microperimetry monitors fixation losses as it maps retinal sensitivity. Each stimulus point is indicated by a numerical sensitivity value as well as a "color value," based on a sensitivity scale. The eye-tracking software incorporated into modern microperimetry compensates for the frequent fixation losses of patients with compromised central vision. Additionally, programs can identify the preferred retinal locus (PRL), which is the area of the retina used for eccentric fixation in patients with central foveal vision loss.

INDICATIONS FOR RETINAL MICROPERIMETRY

Retinal microperimetry is not routinely used in clinical practice but is most commonly ordered to characterize patients with low vision secondary to undefined retinal degeneration. In patients without an obvious structural retinal abnormality, microperimetry can identify areas of reduced sensitivity and localize them onto an image of the retina with a high degree of accuracy. The tool is helpful for monitoring sensitivity losses over time. Additionally, for low-vision rehabilitation, the test is essential for identifying any PRLs, which can be used by patients to compensate for

Gologorsky D, Rosen RB, eds.
Principles of Ocular Imaging (pp 149-152).
© 2021 Taylor & Francis Group.

their vision loss and get the most out of their remaining field of vision. New modalities also offer biofeedback fixation training that aims to teach patients to consistently use their new PRL and avoid returning to PRLs in areas of the retina that have suboptimal sensitivity.

How to Interpret Retinal Perimetry

Microperimetry superimposes a detailed map of retinal function over images that demonstrate the geographic organization of retinal structural changes and lesions. This allows the ophthalmologist to correlate structural and functional changes of the retina in a single test. A good first step in retinal perimetry interpretation is to observe the bare image of the fundus, captured with scanning laser or a fundus photograph, for any structural abnormalities. The next step involves evaluating the map of retinal sensitivity, identifying areas of decreased sensitivity. Some measures of fixation stability will also be presented. This measure should be evaluated to assess that the test has not been compromised by excessive fixation losses. Lastly, many modern software programs also include identification of the patient's preferred area of fixation. If a patient has lost foveal vision, this PRL will occur outside of the fovea. Identification of this PRL is important in training patients in low-vision clinics to leverage what remaining vision they may have.

Common Terms

- *Sensitivity*: the threshold at which retinal photoreceptors can sense light of a particular luminance level

- *Luminance*: a quantitative measure of light intensity per unit area of a stimulus

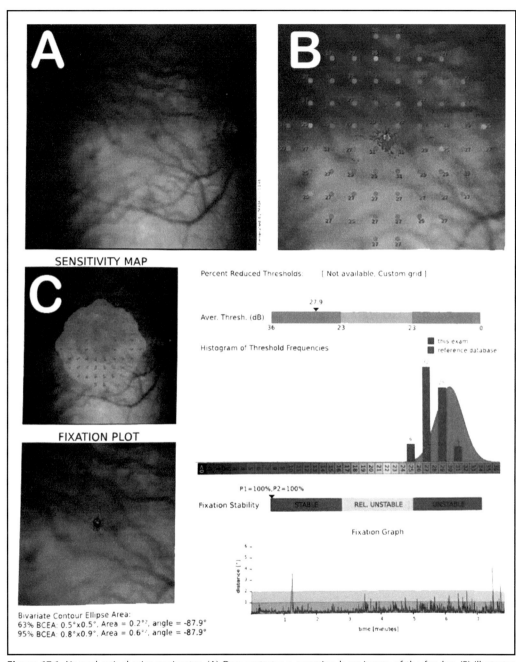

Figure 17-1. Normal retinal microperimetry. (A) Demonstrates a scanning laser image of the fundus. (B) Illustrates sensitivity markers overlaid onto the scanning laser imaging. (C) Corresponds to the color stimulus intensity threshold.

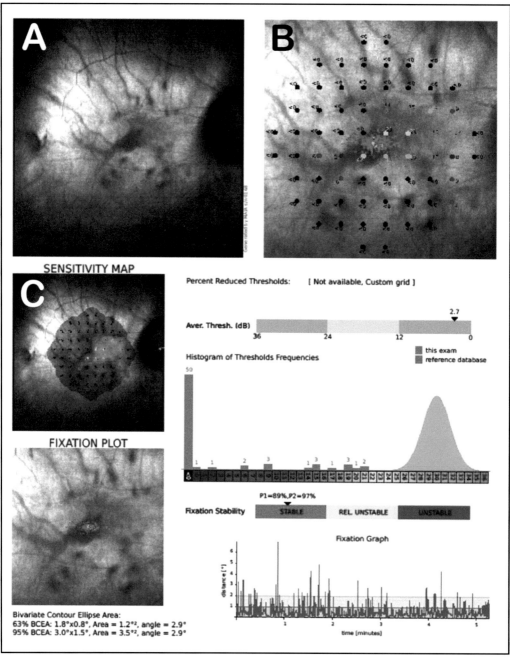

Figure 17-2. Retinal microperimetry in a patient with choroideremia. (A) Demonstrates a scanning laser image of the fundus. (B) Illustrates sensitivity markers overlaid onto the scanning laser imaging, indicating the retinal sensitivity at particular locations throughout the fundus. (C) Corresponds to the color stimulus intensity threshold. Black dots demonstrate areas of complete loss of retinal perception, while the red dots represent diminished response. Green indicates normal retinal sensitivity as compared to a reference database of normal patients. The fixation stability spectrum indicates the degree of patient fixation. Modern microperimetry often includes eye-tracking software as many of these patients have low vision and trouble with fixation.

18

RETINAL ULTRASONOGRAPHY

Daniel Gologorsky, MD, MBA
Yale Fisher, MD

While the topic of extraocular and orbital ultrasonography was presented earlier in this book (Chapter 4), the following brief text will review how ultrasonography works and will provide clinical examples that focus on intraocular indications for ultrasonography.

Ultrasonography is the essential imaging modality for structures of the eye and orbit that are obscured to the examiner. It provides an intraocular evaluation when no view to the fundus is possible and can help assess structures of the orbit including the extraocular muscles. It can also be used in instances where the patient's eyes are difficult to examine, such as nystagmus.

Ophthalmic ultrasonography, similar to ultrasonography elsewhere in the body, entails pulse-echo technology with high frequency sound waves emitted from a handheld transducer probe, where returning echoes are recorded and displayed in real time on a monitor. Clinical ultrasound devices are mobile and include three parts: the transducer probe, a signal processor, and a display monitor. Most commercial ophthalmic ultrasound devices employ 10 MHz transducer probes, although higher resolution devices (20 to 50 MHz) exist, albeit at the expense of tissue penetration.

When performing an orbital ultrasound, the handheld probe is gently placed against the eyelid or sclera using a sound-coupling agent, such as methylcellulose, and the transducer is pointed toward the relevant tissue while viewing the monitor for guidance. Two display modes are utilized: the A-scan mode reveals information about the reflectivity of a particular tissue, in the form of vertical deflections from a baseline produced by the echoes. The B-scan mode sweeps an arc of A-scans providing a cross-sectional view of a cone of tissue within the eye or orbit. Interpretation of ultrasonography involves studying real-time movie segments and grayscale-intensity characteristics to elicit a three-dimensional mental reconstruction of the structures based upon multiple cross sections.

Gologorsky D, Rosen RB, eds.
Principles of Ocular Imaging (pp 153-159).
© 2021 Taylor & Francis Group.

It is important to be aware that on the ultrasound display, tissues closest to the transducer appear to the left, and those furthest appear on the right. Every handheld transducer has a notch or a dot at its barrel. This marks the top of the image displayed and the initial position for each sector scan. One can examine the entire globe in five simple maneuvers: four dynamic quadrant views and one static longitudinal cut through the macula and optic nerve. The quadrants are labelled as if a clock were superimposed onto the globe: T12 superior, T6 inferior, and T3 and T6 temporal or nasal, depending on the eye being examined. During the ultrasound, the patient should look in the direction of the quadrant being evaluated.

The following clinical examples illustrate the application of ultrasonography for various intra-ocular indications.

Figure 18-1. B-scan ultrasound of a normal eye and orbit.

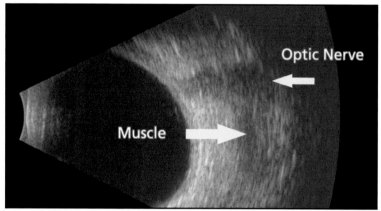

Figure 18-2. An ultrasound demonstrating floaters (arrow) with an attached vitreous face.

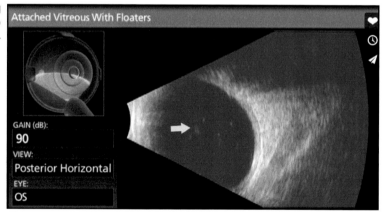

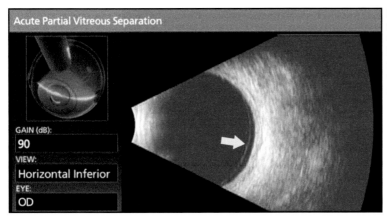

Figure 18-3. An ultrasound demonstrating a partial posterior vitreous detachment in a patient with acute new floaters (arrow). The vitreous gel is not separated from the posterior pole in all cuts.

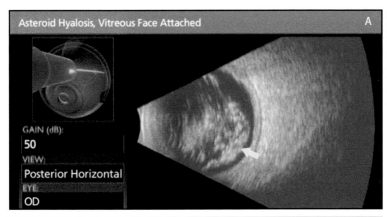

Figure 18-4. (A) Asteroid hyalosis is evident as scintillating hyperechoic debris in the vitreous cavity (arrow). The vitreous face is still attached to the retina. (B) There is clear evidence of an early vitreous detachment (arrow).

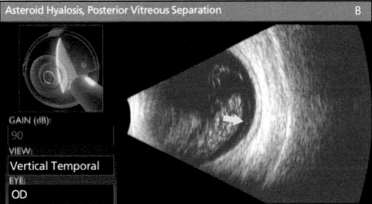

Figure 18-5. (A) An ultrasound image of a choroidal detachment (arrows). (B) If the two opposing choroidals touch (arrow), they are referred to as "kissing choroidals." The retina is attached in both images.

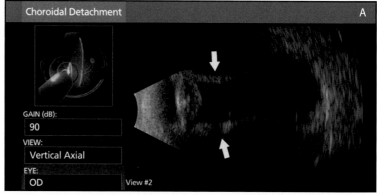

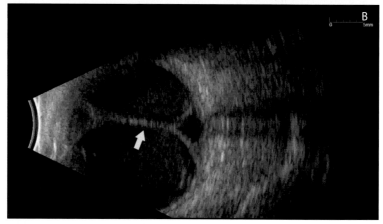

Figure 18-6. An ultrasound image demonstrating a posterior vitreous detachment (yellow arrow) with a final tenuous attachment to the optic nerve (green arrow).

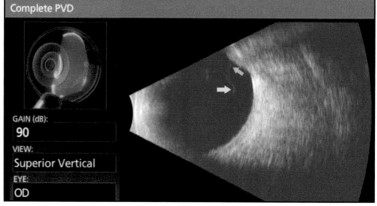

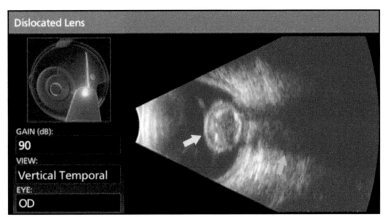

Figure 18-7. A traumatic dislocation of the crystalline lens, captured on ultrasound. The lens is resting on the retina (yellow arrow) and casts a long shadow (green arrow).

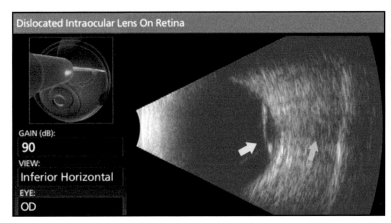

Figure 18-8. A dislocated intraocular lens resting on the inferior retinal surface (yellow arrow) casting a lighter shadow (green arrow) than in the previous example.

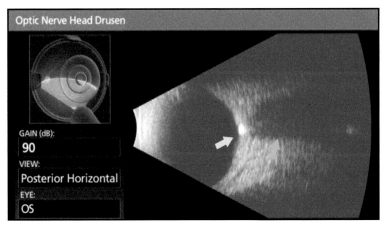

Figure 18-9. Ultrasonography can be particularly useful in evaluating anomalous optic nerves. Optic nerve head drusen demonstrate a classic hyperechoic pattern (yellow arrow) with posterior signal blockage (green arrow).

Figure 18-10. A retinal flap tear captured on ultrasound. (A) The vitreous is adherent to the edge of retinal flap (white arrow). (B) The tear (yellow arrow) is associated with a complete posterior vitreous detachment (green arrow). (C) The retinal tear is associated with vitreous hemorrhage (red arrow).

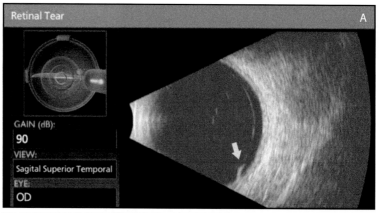

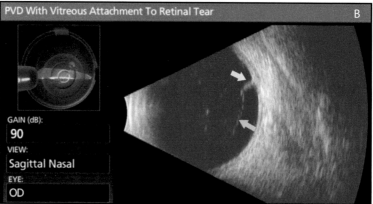

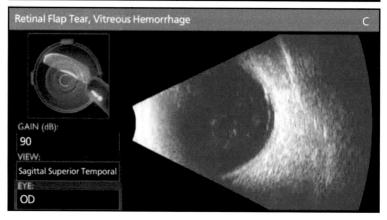

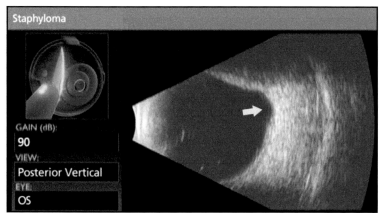

Figure 18-11. An excavation at the posterior pole, consistent with a posterior staphyloma, is evident on ultrasound.

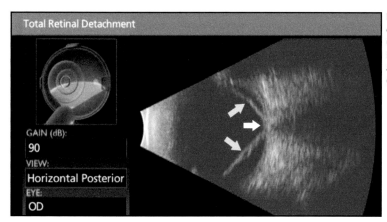

Figure 18-12. A total retinal detachment is evident on ultrasound (yellow arrows). Note that the retina remains attached at the optic nerve (white arrow).

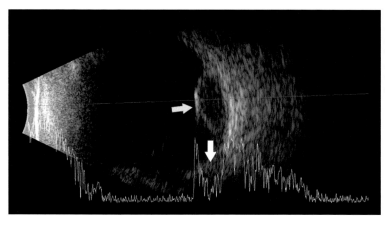

Figure 18-13. A B-scan ultrasound image capturing a choroidal mass (yellow arrow) with an overlaying A-scan showing low internal reflectivity (white arrow) consistent with a choroidal melanoma.

Note: All the figures in this chapter are reprinted with permission from Dr. Yale Fisher's website https://ophthalmicedge.org.

19

ELECTROPHYSIOLOGY OF VISION

Alessandra Bertolucci, MD

The purpose of electrophysiology of vision (EV) is to measure and quantify the electrical properties of the retinal photoreceptors, retinal pigment epithelium (RPE), and visual cortex. Electrophysiologic tests measure voltage changes across the retina, RPE, and visual cortex in response to a light stimulus. These tests are very valuable imaging modalities that prove especially helpful in challenging or unusual clinical cases.

The reader should be aware that there are international standards that regulate the EV testing. The standards are set by the International Society of Clinical Electrophysiology of Vision. The standardized tests performed in an EV laboratory include the full-field electroretinogram (ERG), multifocal ERG (mERG), electro-oculogram (EOG), and visually evoked potential (VEP).

As a review, there are two types of photoreceptors in the eye, rods and cones. The rod cells comprise the vast majority, with over 100 million rod photoreceptors per eye. The rod cells enable one to see in the dark. The cone cells, fewer than 10 million per eye and largely concentrated in the macula, enable high-resolution and color vision.

As an overview, an ERG measures the electrical output of the eye's photoreceptors and produces a single wave that represents the summation of the activities of all the rods, cones, and mixed rod-cone responses to a transient light stimulus. On the other hand, the mERG measures macular function only, and thus records only cone responses. An mERG is evoked by a large series of stimuli, and a computer generates a regional map of macular function. Unlike an ERG or mERG, an EOG measures only the change in potential of the RPE layer, based upon a period of dark adaptation, followed by a phase of light adaptation. VEP, in contrast, measures the electrical activity of the visual cortex; an electrical signal is evoked by a light stimulus and is quantified for each eye. The following section reviews each of these four EV testing modalities in more detail.

Gologorsky D, Rosen RB, eds.
Principles of Ocular Imaging (pp 161-171).
© 2021 Taylor & Francis Group.

ELECTRORETINOGRAM

The full-field ERG is a test that measures photoreceptor function. The setup involves two electrodes; one is a measuring electrode that is in contact with the cornea or conjunctiva, and the other is a reference electrode connected to the lids. In performing an ERG, the patient must first be dilated and should then be dark adapted by being placed in a dark environment for 15 minutes in order to maximize rod sensitivity to light stimuli. This first step of an ERG is done under dark, or scotopic conditions. The initial scotopic testing measures the rods' responses exclusively with a single dim light stimulating both eyes at the same time. The dim stimulus is subthreshold for the cone system, thereby isolating the rod response. The second step entails a single large flash of light, which generates a large response with a negative a-wave followed by a larger, positive b-wave. As a review, the a-wave represents the electrical activity of the photoreceptors, and the b-wave indicates the Muller cell activity.

The third step of an ERG measures the oscillatory potential of the eye, recorded as wavelets within the ascending limb of the b-wave measured under scotopic condition. The subsequent two steps are performed under photopic condition after a 10 minute light adaptation. The photopic phase of the ERG entails a single flash that generates a mixed response due to contributions from both rod and cone cells. Finally, the last portion of an ERG is called the flicker test, where a rapidly flickering stimulus is generated, which is faster than the rods are able to respond and therefore isolates cone responses exclusively.

An ERG is especially helpful in assessing retinal function in the context of rod or cone dystrophies. Besides serving as a diagnostic modality, it is also useful for serial assessment of the progression of retinal disease. Examples of entities followed using ERG include posterior uveitis such as Birdshot chorioretinopathy, cases of unexplained vision loss, siderosis bulbi, and retinitis sine pigmenti.

MULTIFOCAL ELECTRORETINOGRAM

The mERG measures the electrical activity of the macula. The macula is the central area of the retina which is responsible for color vision and highly discriminating central vision due to its concentration of cone cells. This test also requires the patient to be dilated in advance. There are two electrodes: a recording electrode, which is in contact with the cornea or conjunctiva, and a reference electrode. Each eye is examined independently, starting usually with the best-functioning eye. A macular ERG response is elicited by a large sequence of computer-generated black and white stimuli. The macular response is measured and amplified and is represented by a map of 103 distinct areas of the macula. For each of these sites, there is a wavelet with a specific morphology, amplitude, and timing. The mERG is an important indicator of macular function and has many clinical applications. It is commonly used to help distinguish between macular vs optic nerve etiologies of vision loss, in cases of suspected Plaquenil toxicity, occult maculopathy, or functional vision loss.

ELECTRO-OCULOGRAM

An EOG measures the variation of the RPE potential between dark and light adaptation. The trough generated during the dark adaptation (scotopic phase) is compared to the peak generated during the light phase (photopic phase). Procedurally, the patient must first be dilated for this test, then recording and reference electrodes are placed outside of the eye. The dark-adapted scotopic phase commences, during which the patient is placed in the dark for 15 minutes and is asked to move his or her eyes in various directions for a specific amount of time. This is followed by a photopic phase of similar duration, with the same eye movements and timing. The ratio of the photopic potential trough (top of light rise) to the scotopic potential (lowest point) is referred to as the Arden ratio. A normal Arden ratio is above 1.85, and any value below 1.65 is pathologic (with values between 1.65 and 1.85 concerning for abnormal). EOGs are best used for the evaluation of RPE dystrophies, pattern dystrophies, and Best's disease.

VISUALLY EVOKED POTENTIAL

A VEP measures a patient's response to a light source in a chessboard or grid-like pattern. Two check sizes are used to challenge the macula: the larger is a 1-degree stimulus, which is followed by the smaller 15-minute stimulus. The electrical signal is measured through recording and reference electrodes on the scalp at the occipital region of the skull. One eye at a time, the patient looks at the stimulus and the response is measured. The large positive wave response is called P100 because it is recorded at 100 milliseconds. There are some variations of this pattern related to different types of stimuli (checkerboards of various shapes and different contrasts). A VEP recording is reliable and very helpful, especially when comparing the two eyes. VEPs are very important in the evaluation of optic neuropathies of various etiologies.

Figure 19-1. Normal ERG printout depicting five waveforms for each eye. The top three readings were taken under scotopic conditions and the bottom two reflect photopic conditions. The top waveform reflects an exclusive rod response. In the middle, one is used to look at the small wavelets that represent small oscillatory potentials, reflecting the activity of the inner retina and amacrine cells. While it may be used as a measure of ischemia, it has limited value in most clinical settings. The bottom window shows the rapid (30 Hz) flicker stimulus which exclusively reflects the cone response.

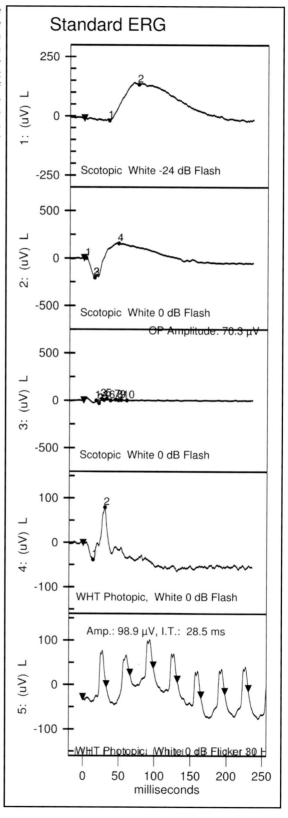

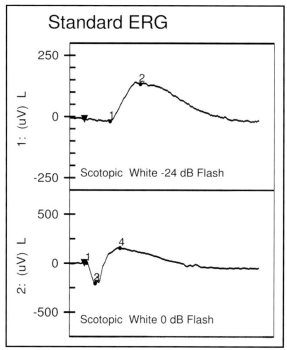

Figure 19-2. Scotopic ERG. The top box waveform reflects a pure rod response. The EV response occurs within the first 100 milliseconds, with an initial flat line reflecting positively with a large b-wave. The downward fall of the wave represents an eyeblink. The second box, representing a single flash under scotopic conditions, is the largest response one can obtain from the retina with a mixed rod and cone response. It demonstrates an initial flat line with a downward inflecting a-wave, followed by a large positive b-wave.

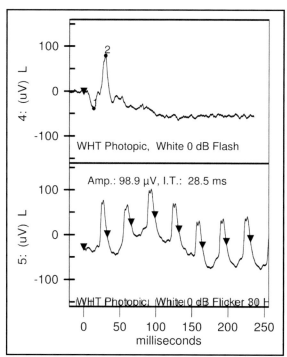

Figure 19-3. Normal single flash under photopic conditions (top box) and normal response to the flicker stimulus (bottom box). The eye is light adapted for 10 minutes, and then experiences a bright flash. This principally stimulates cones, with a small contribution of rod responses as well. The waveform demonstrates a single a-wave followed by a large b-wave. The bottom box is called an automated "flicker stimulus" at 30 Hz, so there is a very rapid response. The peak of the response correlates to a cone-only response. It is a quantifiable and repeatable response.

Figure 19-4. Example of a flat ERG consistent with laboratory confirmed Leber's congenital amaurosis due to an RPE65 gene mutation. Overall there is virtually no cone or rod response. There is an absent rod response in the top box and a minimal residual cone function in the bottom box.

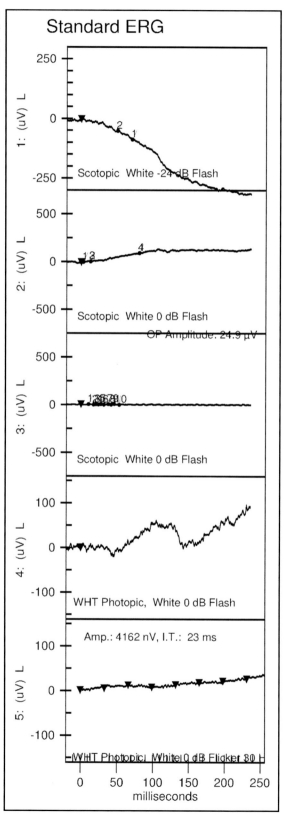

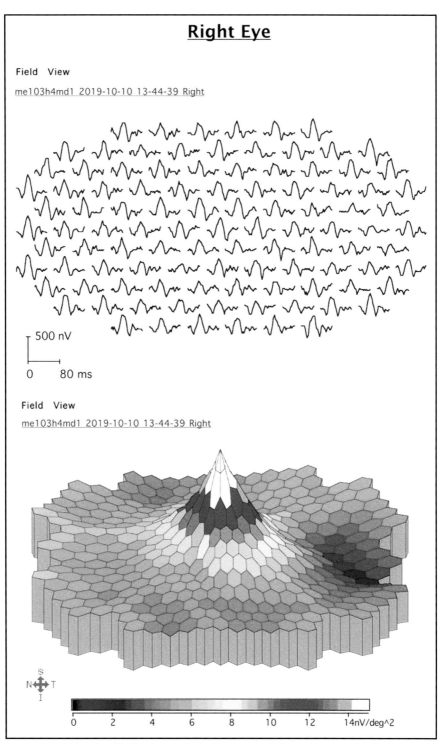

Figure 19-5. Normal mERG. This test evaluates 30 degrees of the macula over 103 distinct areas. A computerized report is generated where actual wavelets themselves are represented over the macula with a three-dimensional rendition based on the amplitude of responses. The highest amplitudes are demonstrated in the center of the macula where cone cells are most concentrated.

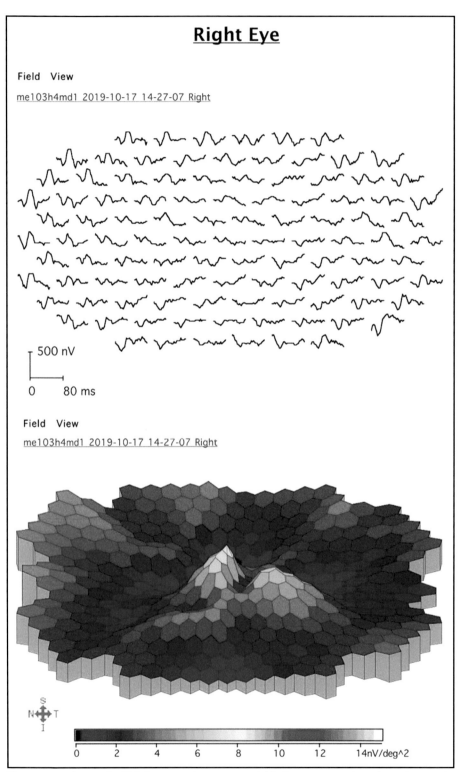

Figure 19-6. Abnormal mERG demonstrating non-recordable flat responses throughout the macula, with poor responses in the periphery (denoted by green and yellow). This particular case represents an advanced Plaquenil (hydroxychloroquine) toxicity.

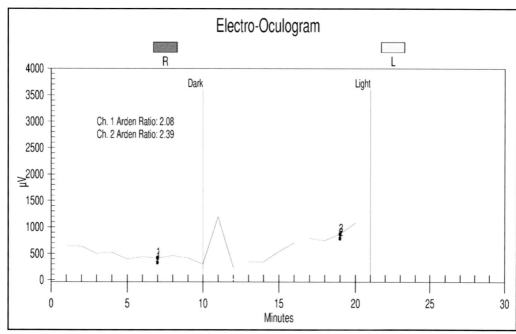

Figure 19-7. Normal EOG. The ratio of the peak to the trough is the Arden ratio.

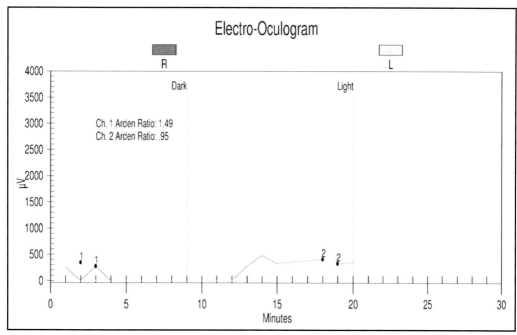

Figure 19-8. Abnormal EOG with an Arden ratio of less than 1.65.

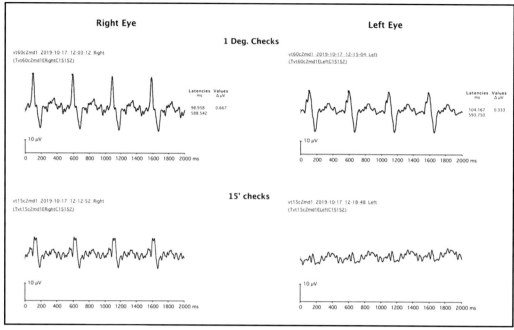

Figure 19-9. Normal VEP. Normal P 100 response to 1-degree and 15-minute stimulus in the right eye. In the left eye the P 100 is delayed for the 1-degree stimulus size and barely visible for the 15-minute check size, compatible with an optic neuritis.

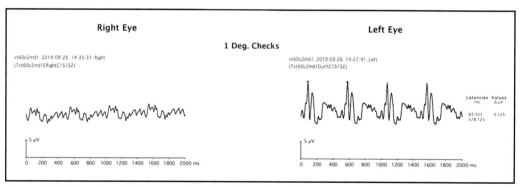

Figure 19-10. There is no P100 response from the right eye for the larger and smaller check sizes. There is a normal P100 in the left eye for the larger and smaller check sizes. These results are consistent with a right optic neuropathy.

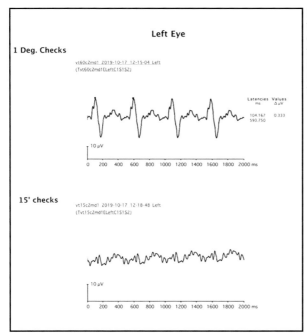

Figure 19-11. VEP showing normal timing (P100) to the larger signal check size (1-degree), but demonstrating delayed timing and smaller amplitude signals when challenged with the smaller (15-degree) check size. This suggests that the macula cannot discriminate the smaller signals; the pattern is consistent with a maculopathy.

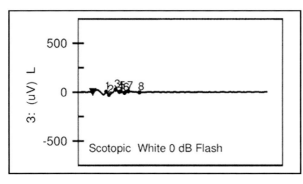

Figure 19-12. Electronegative response. After a single flash under scotopic conditions, this patient demonstrates a normal a-wave, although the b-wave does not recover to the baseline. The patient with this electronegative response suffered from congenital stationary night blindness.

Section IV
Glaucoma

Section Editor
Stephen Moster, MD

20

Visual Fields in Glaucoma

Stephen Moster, MD
Cindy X. Zheng, MD
Michael M. Lin, MD

Visual field testing is an important diagnostic tool for the evaluation of retinal, neurological, and optic nerve diseases. Changes in the visual field reflect defects in the visual field pathway and their proper interpretation are paramount for making correct diagnoses. The most common use of visual field tests is for the detection and monitoring of glaucoma. Patients often undergo multiple tests per year since assessing subtle progression on physical exam and other testing modalities can be challenging.

THE HILL OF VISION

The eye can see roughly 60 degrees superiorly and nasally, 70 degrees inferiorly, and 100 degrees temporally. Visual field testing traditionally concentrates on the central 30 degrees due to the retina's variable ability to detect dim lights in the periphery. Visual sensitivity is greatest in the fovea and decreases gradually in the periphery. A graphic depiction of the eye's sensitivity appears as a "Hill of Vision." With age, the gradual reduction in sensitivity to light lowers the profile of the "Hill."

Gologorsky D, Rosen RB, eds.
Principles of Ocular Imaging (pp 175-184).
© 2021 Taylor & Francis Group.

Goldmann Kinetic Perimetry

An early form of the visual field testing utilizing kinetic perimetry became standardized as Goldmann perimetry. This involves moving a stimulus of varying size from the periphery inward until the patient signals when they can first detect the stimulus. The hill of vision can be mapped out based on the size and brightness of each stimulus. Defects in the field are recognized when standard stimuli are not appreciated in a meridian, or require larger or brighter test objects to be seen. Goldmann visual fields are time consuming, operator dependent, and difficult to reproduce, and are therefore no longer used as the main perimetry tool.

Testing Strategies

Automated static perimetry is currently the most commonly used platform. The stimuli are static, meaning that targets appear and disappear in different areas of the patient's visual field, but do not move. This provides a more reproducible and standardized testing method with quantifiable results. The Humphrey Visual Field (Carl Zeiss Meditec, Inc) is the most popular machine in the United States followed by the Octopus (Haag-Streit Diagnostics) instrument. Traditionally, static perimetry relied on a full-threshold strategy to measure the retina's sensitivity. This involved multiple adjustments in light sensitivity at each point until the dimmest stimulus was appreciated. The Humphrey visual field currently relies on the Swedish Interactive Threshold Algorithm (SITA), which uses a mathematical model based on sensitivities to surrounding locations, age matched controls, and trends in visual field changes in glaucoma patients. This algorithm requires fewer stimuli to determine the hill of vision and has reduced test times by half (compared to full threshold testing), which has produced more reliable test results.

Stimulus Size, Luminance, and Testing Algorithms

Traditional target sizes are derived from the Goldman "stimulus size III" and measure 4 mm^2. The second most commonly used target size is 64 mm^2 and is referred to as the Goldman "stimulus size V." This larger stimulus is often reserved for patients with poor visual acuity or diffusely-depressed fields. Stimulus size V exams are often longer and do not include comparisons to the normal population (global indices) since the SITA and STATPAC software is based on Stim III only.

The traditional 24-2 test measures 54 spots. The test measures 24 degrees in each direction except for nasally (which measures out to 30 degrees), since glaucomatous changes often begin in this area. As glaucomatous damage advances, the visual field becomes constricted, and often the only points in the center are visualized. Switching to a 10-2 threshold (which measures 68 spots in the central 10 degrees) allows for more reliable testing of progression in these patients and in any patient with paracentral defects.

Reliability Indices

Visual field testing demands good cooperation and attention from the patient. Without proper focus, dim stimuli will go unnoticed and fields will appear worse. Conversely, anxious patients may press the response trigger even when a stimulus is not presented. Therefore, there are four reliability indices on a SITA field: fixation losses, false negative errors, false positive errors, and a gaze tracker.

The perimeter maps the blind spot and periodically a light signal is sent in that area. If a patient perceives a stimulus in their blind spot, their fixation has drifted and it is considered a fixation loss. Fixation losses are the least important of the reliability indices and should not be weighted heavily if other parameters are within normal limits. An adjunct measurement is the gaze tracker at the bottom of the printout. The cornea is followed and every time the eye moves there is an uptick noted. If the machine cannot tell whether the patient moved, there is a downward bar displayed. Typically, there will be more ticks in either direction during longer exams, indicating variability in the patient's attention.

False positive errors are very important for determining if a field is uninterpretable. The machine makes a sound as if displaying a light, but without actually presenting a light. Anxious patients may click the trigger when they hear a sound, or randomly when very dim lights are presented even though they are not seen. This results in greater sensitivities and superhuman threshold values. Interpreting a test with high false positives may lead to a false sense of reassurance while missing defects or progression.

False negatives represent fatigue and poor attention. The patient has stopped responding and misses brighter stimuli in areas that were previously thresholded. This often results in generalized depression and a field that may look worse than the true defect. Note however that later in disease, as defects increase in depth and size, higher false negatives are expected due to the variability in ganglion cells' perception of light.

Deviation Maps

The total deviation plot shows the amount of deviation of each point in the visual field from age-matched normals. The graph generated below the visual field shows the statistical significance of each point. Since peripheral variability is expected, a peripheral defect on the total deviation plot may seem important, but will not register as statistically significant compared to controls.

The pattern deviation map uncovers glaucomatous defects hidden by generalized depression from media opacities. This map uses the seventh most sensitive point in the visual field and sets that point as the new zero. Any defects deeper than that threshold value are displayed with negative numbers and their statistical significance is displayed below.

Global Indices

Mean deviation is an average deviation of each spot from age-matched normals. It is derived from the total deviation plot and is centrally weighted, since central defects are more reproducible and clinically important. It is affected by media opacities such as dry eye, vitreous hemorrhage, and cataracts. The mean deviation should improve with correction of media opacity (ie, cataract surgery) and progressively worsens in uncontrolled glaucoma.

Pattern standard deviation (PSD) is a measure of focal loss within visual field defects and is not influenced by generalized depression. As a defect becomes more broad or deep, the PSD increases. Eventually, as greater amounts of the field become "universally" involved, defects are less focal and the PSD may decrease, signifying worsening glaucoma.

The glaucoma hemifield test involves a comparison of defects in the superior and inferior fields. This is useful since glaucoma often progresses asymmetrically in one hemifield before the other is involved. This is often sensitive for early loss since the patient's own minor defects are compared to the other hemifield as a control.

Progression Analysis

The Guided Progression Analysis is derived from the Manifest Glaucoma Trial. The first two visual fields are used as a baseline. Once a baseline is established, each point on follow up visual fields is compared to the baseline values. If a point has a statistically significant change, an open triangle is displayed at that point. If the same defect is present on two tests, then a half-filled triangle is displayed. A filled triangle represents confirmed worsening seen on three tests. If at least three points are consecutively worse on two exams, an alert of "possible progression" is displayed. If seen on a third test, "likely progression" is displayed.

The visual field index (VFI) is a percentage value (1% to 100%) assigned to visual fields based on age and visual function compared to normals. The value is based on the pattern deviation and relies on central points due to peripheral variability. The VFI graph is a trend analysis of the percentage values and determines the rate of change as well as its statistical significance. The VFI requires multiple fields in order to determine an accurate trend.

REPEAT TESTING

Changes in sensitivity at one or more clustered points should not be taken lightly. Often true defects that are confirmed on repeat testing represent significant ganglion cell loss in that particular region of the retina. However, a fluctuation in test sensitivity is common, and defects that appear glaucomatous often resolve on repeat testing. These artifacts can be misleading and testing should always be repeated if worsening occurs. A test may be overall reliable, though defects may appear in one area if the patient loses focus. This was established in the Ocular Hypertension Treatment Study which showed that 85.9% of visual fields that appeared glaucomatous resolved with repeat testing.

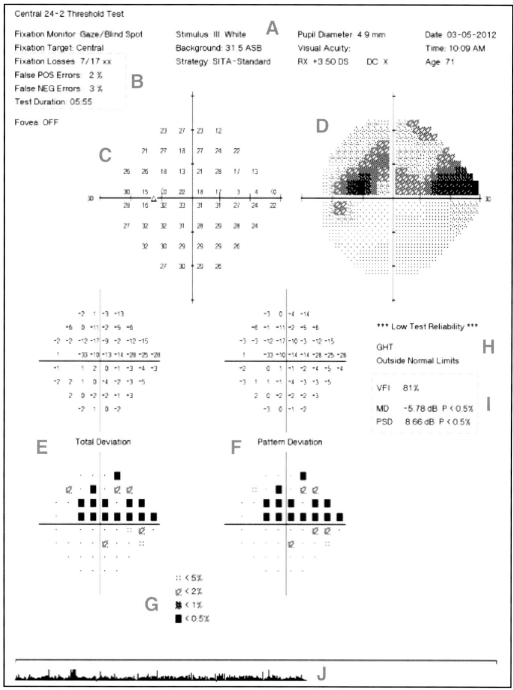

Figure 20-1. Single field analysis. (A) Patient information and testing type. (B) Reliability indices. (C) Test results measured in decibels at each location. Higher numbers represent visualization of very dim stimuli. A number zero means the patient cannot see the brightest stimulus. All other printout information is derived from these measurements. (D) Grayscale. (E) Total deviation: variance from age-matched normals on top, likelihood each abnormal measurement occurred by chance below. (F) Pattern deviation: correction of total deviation by subtracting all points based on the depression of the seventh most sensitive value (top) and the likelihood the remaining defects occurred by chance (bottom). (G) Statistical significance of each point. (H) Glaucoma hemifield test. (I) Global indices: visual field index, mean deviation, and pattern standard deviation. (J) Gaze tracker.

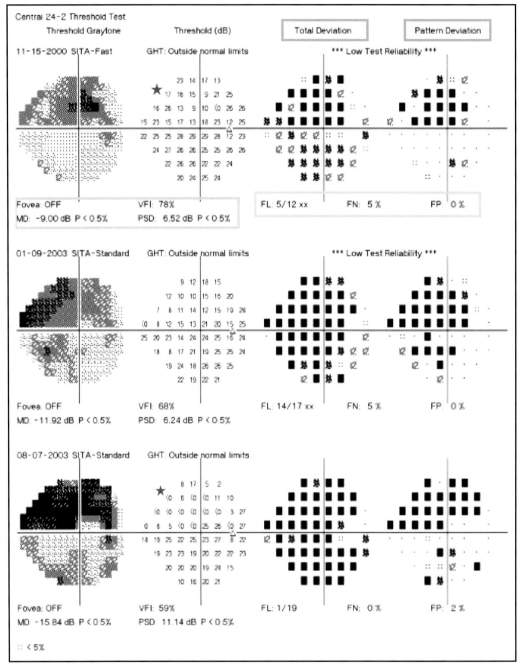

Figure 20-2. Overview from multiple fields from a different patient. Includes grayscale, threshold results, total deviation, and pattern deviation (red boxes). Reliability indices (green box) and global indices (blue box) are listed beneath each exam. Notice the worsening threshold values over time (red stars) and worsening global indices.

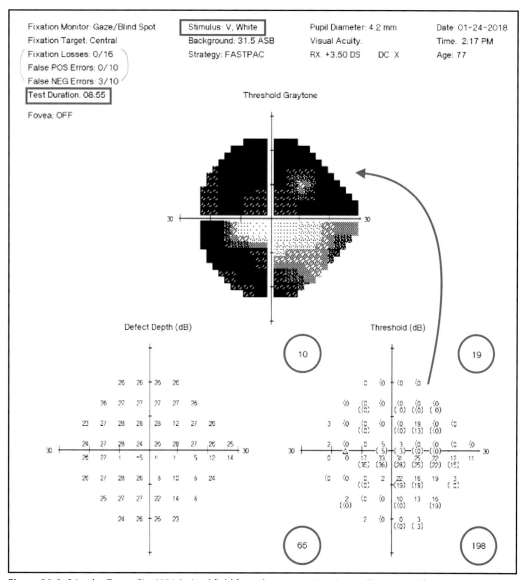

Figure 20-3. Stimulus Target Size V 24-2 visual field from the same patient/eye as Figure 20-1. The patient had severe worsening of glaucoma over time, now requiring a Stim V due to severe generalized depression on Stim III. The Stim V testing strategy is not SITA like in traditional Stim III visual fields and lacks comparisons to age-matched normals. Therefore, the printout does not have the same deviation plots or global indices. The grayscale is presented on the top and the threshold values are presented in the left lower quadrant. The sum total of threshold values for each quadrant are presented (blue circles), which gives an overall sense of visual sensitivity that is fairly easy to follow over time. This field has significant depression and constriction (red arrow), which makes determining progression difficult. Therefore, the testing strategy was switched to a 10-2 (Figure 20-4). Note the longer test length without the SITA algorithm.

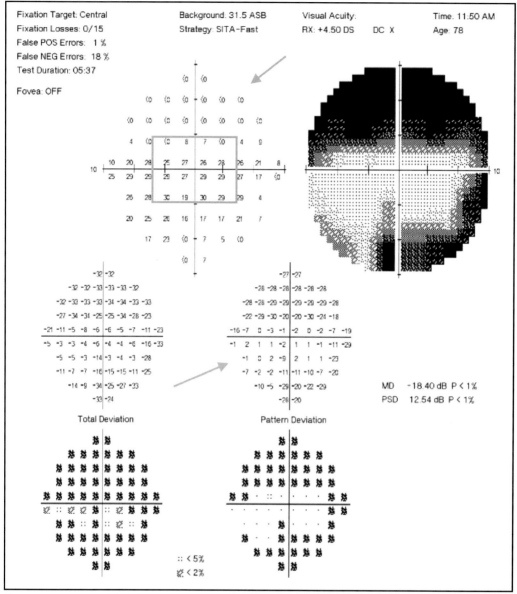

Figure 20-4. 10-2 Visual field from the same patient as Figures 20-1 and 20-3. This exam focuses on the central 10 degrees. The points tested are separated by only 2 degrees as compared to 6 degrees on a 24-2. The central 10-degree region is only measured by four total test points on a 24-2 (one paracentral point in each quadrant). In the 24-2 exam (Figure 20-3), there appears to be dense defects centrally, though the 10-2 shows there are points that have yet to become affected from glaucoma (within blue rectangle). The blue arrow shows that the glaucomatous defects are not only diffuse but very deep; this patient is unable to see the brightest stimuli superiorly. The red arrow shows the test points that will be followed for progression.

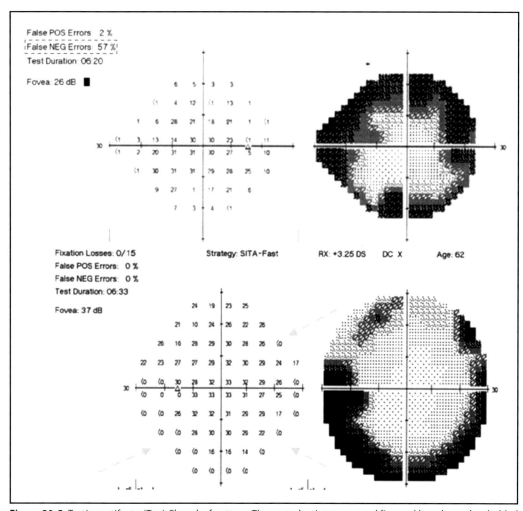

Figure 20-5. Testing artifacts. (Top) Cloverleaf pattern. The central points are tested first and have been thresholded appropriately. This patient lost attention early on. Note the high false negatives. (Bottom) Rim artifact. Notice that defects are limited to the periphery and are very dense (0 dB, arrows). This is a result of the rim from the lens placed in front of the eye blocking the light stimuli. This is also seen when a patient's head leans slightly back from the forehead rest.

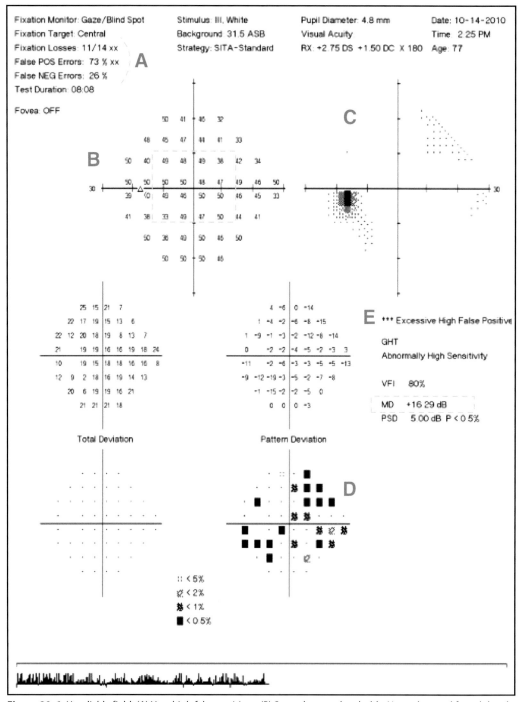

Figure 20-6. Unreliable field. (A) Very high false positives. (B) Super-human thresholds. Normal central foveal thresholds are typically in the mid 30s. (C) Grayscale shows "white out." (D) Pattern deviation shows a "reverse cataract." (E) The hemifield test mentions "excessive high false positives." Note the mean deviation is 16 dB greater than normals (blue rectangle).

21

OPTICAL COHERENCE TOMOGRAPHY IN GLAUCOMA

Michael M. Lin, MD
Cindy X. Zheng, MD
Stephen Moster, MD

BACKGROUND

Optical coherence tomography (OCT) is a noninvasive, noncontact imaging technique that is commonly used in the diagnosis and management of glaucoma. It was first primarily used to assess retinal nerve fiber layer (RNFL) thickness and optic nerve head parameters; macular retinal ganglion cell layer thickness has recently become a useful metric as well. Time-domain OCT was first described in 1991 and became commercially available in 1996. The technology improved rapidly and was quickly replaced by spectral-domain OCT (SD-OCT), which was first described in 2003. SD-OCT is also called Fourier-domain OCT, or video-rate OCT, and has a resolution of 5 to 7 μm.

OCT is commonly described as similar to ultrasound imaging except that light is used instead of sound. First, light is passed through a beam splitter and goes toward the eye and a reference mirror. The reflectance pattern from the light that reaches the eye varies based on the reflectivity of the ocular tissues. Next, the interference patterns of reflected light coming back from the eye and from the reference mirror are combined to produce an image. OCT machines have automated segmentation algorithms that identify the different layers of the retina in these images, including the RNFL, which thins in glaucoma due to loss of retinal ganglion cells. OCT provides an opportunity to visualize the microscopic structural changes that may precede visual field changes in glaucoma, and is useful for monitoring patients with ocular hypertension or mild glaucoma instead of frequent visual fields.

Gologorsky D, Rosen RB, eds.
Principles of Ocular Imaging (pp 185-197).
© 2021 Taylor & Francis Group.

There are four commonly used commercially available OCT machines in the United States:

1. Cirrus High-Definition (HD) OCT (Carl Zeiss Meditec, Inc)
2. Spectralis SD-OCT (Heidelberg Engineering Inc)
3. RTVue100 (Optovue, Inc)
4. 3D OCT-1000 and 3D OCT-2000 (Topcon Corporation)

These machines are comparable in their ability to help clinicians diagnose and monitor glaucoma. Each has unique scan patterns, segmentation algorithms, data display formats, and progression analysis methods. Because of these variations, RNFL measurements are not interchangeable between machines. Cirrus, in particular, reports slightly lower thicknesses than other machines.

POTENTIAL PITFALLS

When evaluating a patient's OCT, after confirming that the image is from the correct patient, it is important to check signal strength and quality of the test (Figure 21-1). Signal strength scores of less than 7 of 10 for Cirrus, 30 to 45 of 100 for RTVue, 15 of 40 for Spectralis, and 60 of 160 for 3D-OCT 2000 can suggest poor image quality. This can be caused by numerous imaging issues, including but not limited to blinking or eye movement artifacts, intervening posterior vitreous detachment, and opacities of the cornea or lens (Figure 21-2). Other potential sources of poorly interpretable images include optic nerve head edema or vitreous adhesion to the peripapillary macula. Either of these can lead to thicker RNFL measurements that can lure clinicians into thinking that they have "cured" glaucoma. It is critical to inspect the automated segmentation of the retinal layers as the algorithms may misinterpret the anatomy, resulting in incorrectly thin or thick RNFL measurements.

Retinal Nerve Fiber Layer

The most commonly assessed OCT parameter in glaucoma is peripapillary RNFL. The RNFL is composed of axons of retinal ganglion cells, and when these ganglion cells die in glaucoma, the RNFL is lost and becomes thinner (Figure 21-3). This thinning can be captured by OCT with intertest variability of approximately 5 to 10 µm. RNFL thickness is directly measured by automated segmentation of retinal images captured by OCT, followed by measurement of the distance between the internal limiting membrane and RNFL border. What defines the RNFL border is set by the manufacturer of the device, which is why RNFL measurements are not interchangeable between brands of OCT.

The RNFL thickness is measured along a 3.45-mm diameter circle centered on the optic nerve. The values along this circle are plotted on a two-dimensional temporal-superior-nasal-inferior-temporal (TSNIT) map. Composite RNFL thicknesses are plotted by quadrants and clock hours, then compared to a normative database of age-matched controls and displayed on pie chart diagrams that are shaded red, yellow, green, and white to indicate RNFL thinning or thickening. These databases were derived primarily using white adults, so the comparisons may not be valid for children and non-white adults.

While it may be tempting to take a shortcut and review only the overall average RNFL thickness and the color-coded diagrams, it is important to evaluate the TSNIT map because focal thinning may not be wide or thin enough to trigger yellow or red shading, but may be indicative of early focal RNFL loss due to glaucoma (Figure 21-4). Progression can take the form of widening or further thinning of a RNFL defect as well as development of a new defect. Normally aging is expected to reduce average RNFL thickness by 0.5 µm/year, primarily driven by superior and

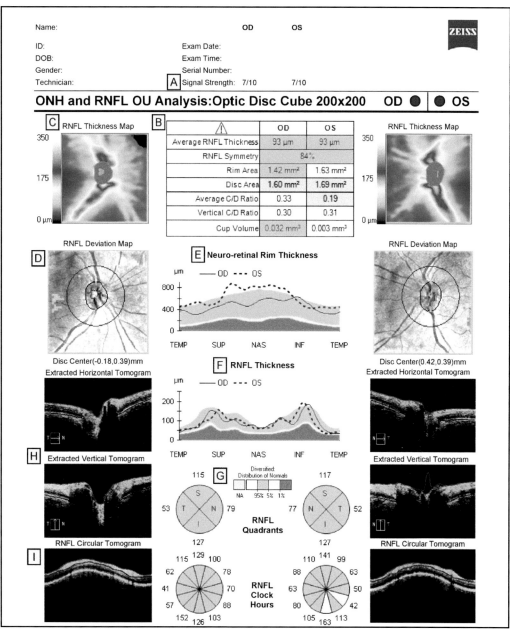

Figure 21-1. OCT RNFL analysis display in a patient without evidence of glaucomatous damage. (A) Signal strength of the scan is displayed at the top of the analysis report. The patient identifying information that would usually be printed in this area has been redacted to preserve confidentiality. (B) Optic nerve head parameters are reported in a table, with shading to indicate how the results compare to a normative database. (C) RNFL thickness map. Superior and inferior poles typically have greatest thickness in normal eyes. (D) RNFL deviation map shows deviation from normative database. (E) Neuro-retinal rim thickness along the purple calculation circle from the RNFL deviation map is plotted for both eyes, with normative data color coded in the background along TSNIT plot. (F) RNFL thickness along the purple calculation circle from the RNFL deviation map is plotted for both eyes, with normative data color-coded in the background along TSNIT plot. (G) RNFL quadrant and clock hour average thicknesses are shaded in comparison to normative data. (H) Horizontal and vertical B-scans through the disc center. Automated segmentation lines are shown. Notice the segmentation error in the left eye vertical tomogram. (I) RNFL calculation circle centered on the optic disc, with automated segmentation lines.

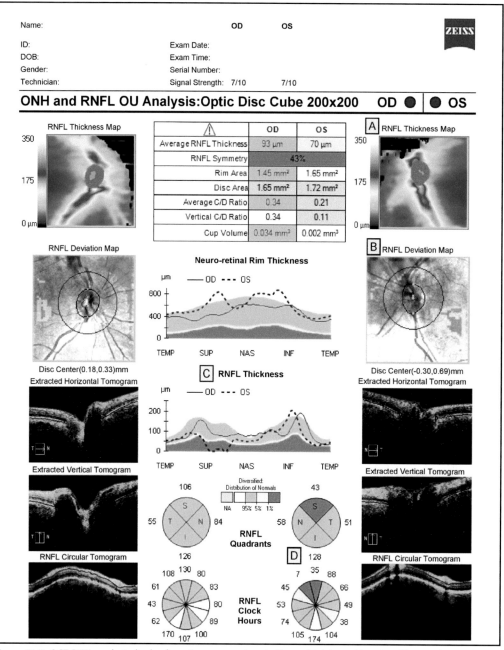

Figure 21-2. OCT RNFL analysis display from the same patient in Figure 21-1, but with a signal loss artifact in the left eye superior RNFL. (A) Black areas at the top of the RNFL thickness map represent areas of signal loss from poor scan quality. (B) Red areas in RNFL deviation map correspond to artifactual thinning due to signal loss. (C) Dotted line representing left eye RNFL thickness dips in superior portion of TSNIT plot. (D) Red superior quadrants and clock hours correspond to artifactual thinning due to signal loss.

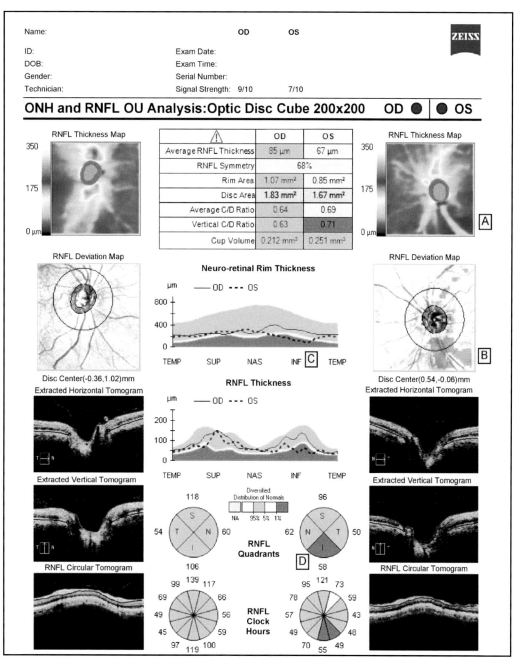

Figure 21-3. OCT RNFL analysis display from a patient with left eye inferior RNFL thinning. (A) Blue shading instead of yellow/orange in the RNFL thickness map. (B) Red shading in the inferior RNFL deviation map. (C) Dotted line representing left eye RNFL thickness dips in the inferior portion of TSNIT plot. (D) Red inferior quadrants and clock hours correspond to inferior RNFL thinning.

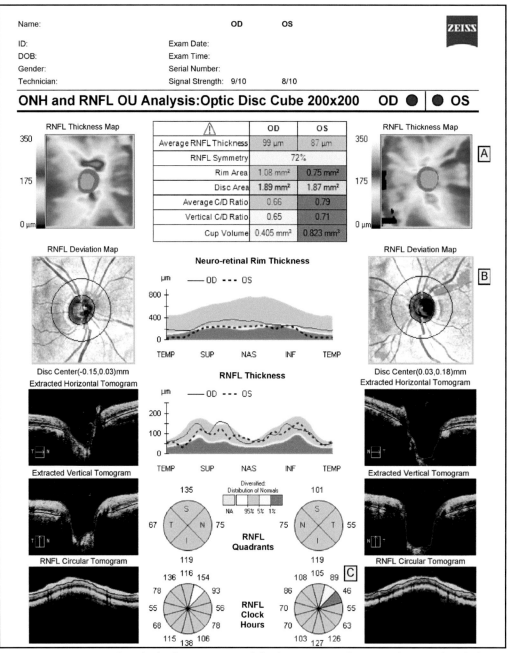

Figure 21-4. OCT RNFL analysis display from a patient with focal superior RNFL loss. Note that even though there is RNFL thinning superiorly, the superior RNFL quadrant remains green because average quadrant thickness has not yet been severely impacted enough by the focal loss to become outside the distribution of normal. (A) Blue shading in the top right part of the image in the superior RNFL bundle demonstrates focal thinning. (B) Red shading in the top right part of the image demonstrates focal thinning. (C) Red and yellow clock hours correspond to RNFL thinning.

inferior RNFL loss of slightly greater than 1 μm/year, typically with minimal nasal and temporal thinning. Therefore, the impact of aging on the RNFL is relatively minor compared to glaucoma. There can also be a "floor effect" in advanced glaucoma causing RNFL thickness to bottom out at approximately 50 μm even though most of the nerve tissue has been lost. This is due to blood vessels, residual glial, and non-neural tissue that will be detected by the OCT machine (Figure 21-5). In these cases, visual fields can be more useful for following end-stage glaucoma.

Macular Retinal Ganglion Cell Layer

More recently, macular retinal ganglion cell layer thickness has become an important parameter in OCT evaluation of glaucoma. A 4- to 10-mm perifoveal area, depending on the machine, is imaged, and automated algorithms report ganglion cell layer thickness as the distance between retinal ganglion cells and the inner plexiform layer (IPL) or the RNFL and the IPL. The ganglion cell layer is measured with the IPL because of the difficulty delineating the border between these layers with current OCT technology. As with RNFL thickness, there is a normative database for ganglion cell layer thickness, and a color-coded scale of thickness map sectors surrounding the fovea is displayed, with yellow and red sectors indicating thinning (Figures 21-6 and 21-7).

Glaucomatous defects on ganglion cell layer maps manifest as arcuate tracks of thinning that stretch from the macula to the optic nerve. Similar to RNFL mapping, ganglion cell layer mapping can suggest progression of glaucoma if the arcuate defect becomes wider or thinner or if a *de novo* area of defect develops. Inferotemporal sector thinning may be the first sign of glaucoma, even before peripapillary RNFL thinning. Significant asymmetry of ganglion cell layer thickness between eyes may also be an important clue to damage.

Some believe that macular OCT of the retinal ganglion cell layer is especially useful in patients with myopic discs because these eyes have thinner RNFL and different RNFL anatomic distribution. The temporal shift of superior and inferior RNFL bundles may make them appear thin compared to reference databases, but the macular OCT may be normal.

When interpreting ganglion cell layer thickness, it is important to evaluate for retinal disease that may make the measurements inaccurate. Conditions such as diabetic macular edema, macular degeneration, retinal vascular occlusions, epiretinal membranes, and vitreomacular traction may alter the measurements or disrupt automated segmentation algorithms.

Optic Nerve Head

OCT can also be a useful supplement to ophthalmoscopy in evaluating the optic nerve head. OCT can quantify optic nerve head size and can outline the optic cup. This allows automated reporting of global metrics such as optic disc area, rim area, vertical cup to disc ratio, and average cup to disc ratio. Studies suggest that the most useful metrics to follow in glaucoma include global rim area, inferior rim area, and vertical cup to disc ratio.

PROGRESSION ANALYSIS

Each OCT machine has its own display output and automated algorithms for reporting progression of glaucomatous damage. In event-based analysis, the display will alert clinicians about potential change when a follow-up image has worsened beyond a threshold that was set using a series of baseline images. In trend-based analysis, the machine reports progression using regression analysis on all images, often highlighting this change by modifying the color of data points along a linear regression line. Yellow or orange data points may indicate first episodes of changes

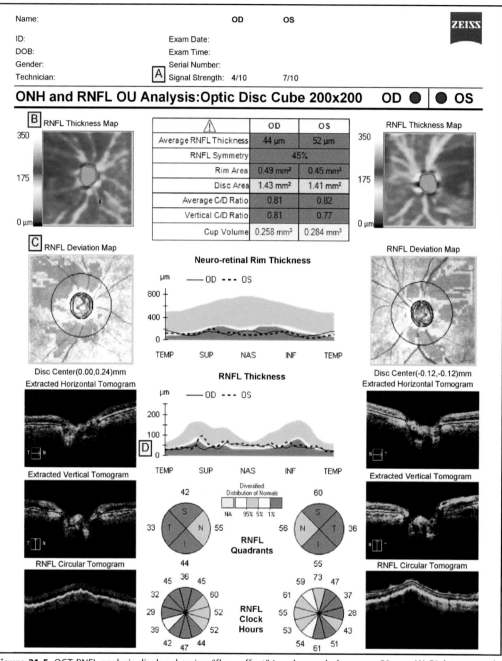

Figure 21-5. OCT RNFL analysis display showing "floor effect" in advanced glaucoma, 50 μm. (A) Right eye results should be interpreted with caution due to poor signal strength, but the left eye image shows better signal strength, building confidence in the OCT measurements. (B) Lack of normal yellow/orange shading superior and inferior to the nerve due to severe RNFL loss. (C) Red shading superior and inferior to the nerve due to severe RNFL loss compared to age-matched controls. (D) RNFL thickness has bottomed out at a thickness of approximately 50 μm because even though most of the RNFL tissue has been lost, there are blood vessels and residual glial and non-neural tissue that will cause OCT machines to report RNFL thickness of approximately 50 μm.

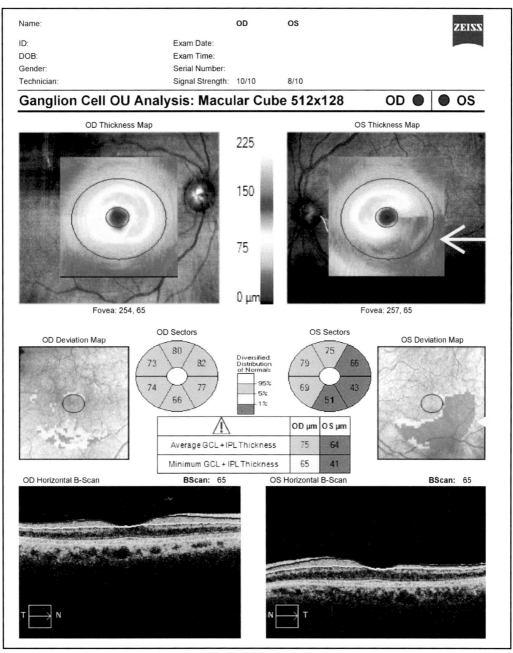

Figure 21-6. OCT ganglion cell analysis display from the same patient in Figure 21-3. Arrows point to where the left eye inferior ganglion cell layer thinning corresponds with the inferior RNFL thinning.

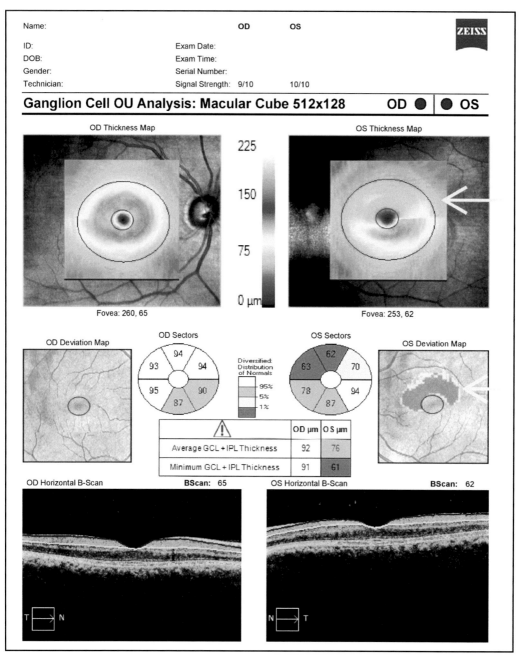

Figure 21-7. OCT ganglion cell analysis display from the same patient in Figure 21-4. Arrows point to where the left eye superior ganglion cell layer thinning corresponds with the superior RNFL thinning.

that exceed test-retest variability, while red spots may indicate changes that have been confirmed on repeated tests (Figure 21-8).

FUTURE DIRECTIONS

While RNFL, macular ganglion cell layer, and optic nerve head imaging are currently the major OCT modalities for diagnosing and monitoring glaucoma, newer reference-plane independent metrics, such as Bruch's membrane opening minimum rim width and minimum distance band, are in development. OCT angiography is also early in clinical use, though it remains unclear whether glaucoma is caused by vascular dropout or merely produces it.

While SD-OCT continues to be the dominant OCT modality, other technologies are on the horizon. Swept-source OCT uses a longer wavelength of light to improve imaging of the lamina cribrosa and choroid. Other machines also in development include polarization sensitive OCT and adaptive optics OCT, which currently remain mostly limited to research purposes instead of widespread clinical use.

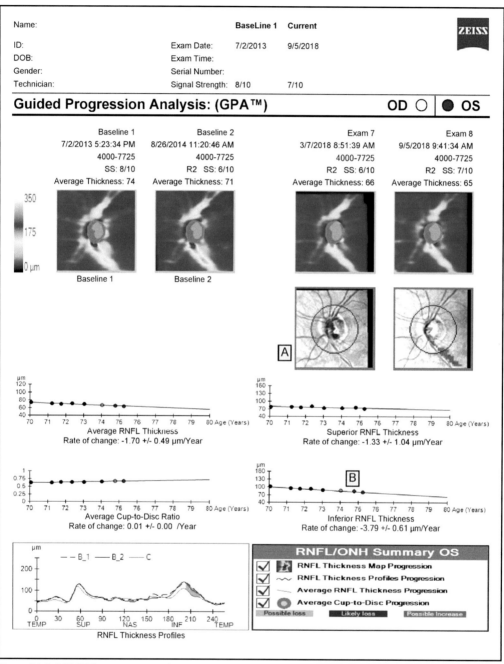

Figure 21-8. OCT RNFL progression analysis in a patient with progressive left eye inferior RNFL loss. (A) RNFL deviation map shows possible inferior thinning in orange and confirmed inferior thinning in red. (B) Orange data points indicate possible RNFL loss, and red data points indicate likely RNFL loss. (*continued*)

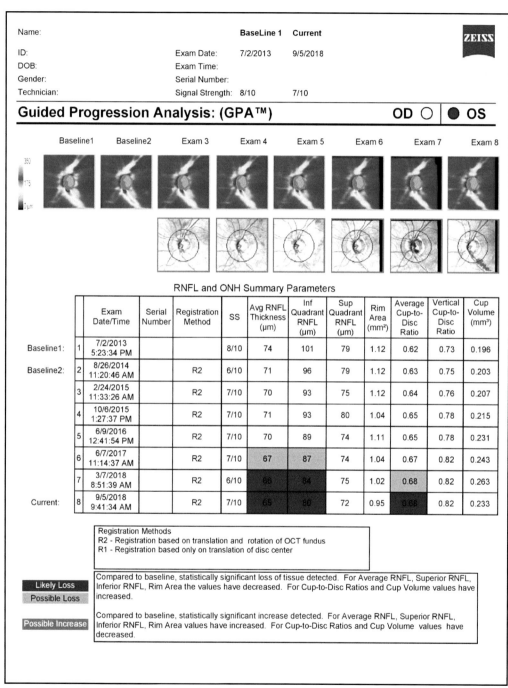

		Exam Date/Time	Serial Number	Registration Method	SS	Avg RNFL Thickness (µm)	Inf Quadrant RNFL (µm)	Sup Quadrant RNFL (µm)	Rim Area (mm²)	Average Cup-to-Disc Ratio	Vertical Cup-to-Disc Ratio	Cup Volume (mm³)
Baseline1:	1	7/2/2013 5:23:34 PM			8/10	74	101	79	1.12	0.62	0.73	0.196
Baseline2:	2	8/26/2014 11:20:46 AM		R2	6/10	71	96	79	1.12	0.63	0.75	0.203
	3	2/24/2015 11:33:26 AM		R2	7/10	70	93	75	1.12	0.64	0.76	0.207
	4	10/6/2015 1:27:37 PM		R2	7/10	71	93	80	1.04	0.65	0.78	0.215
	5	6/9/2016 12:41:54 PM		R2	7/10	70	89	74	1.11	0.65	0.78	0.231
	6	6/7/2017 11:14:37 AM		R2	7/10	67	87	74	1.04	0.67	0.82	0.243
	7	3/7/2018 8:51:39 AM		R2	6/10	68	84	75	1.02	0.68	0.82	0.263
Current:	8	9/5/2018 9:41:34 AM		R2	7/10	65	80	72	0.95	0.68	0.82	0.233

Registration Methods
R2 - Registration based on translation and rotation of OCT fundus
R1 - Registration based only on translation of disc center

Likely Loss
Possible Loss
Possible Increase

Compared to baseline, statistically significant loss of tissue detected. For Average RNFL, Superior RNFL, Inferior RNFL, Rim Area the values have decreased. For Cup-to-Disc Ratios and Cup Volume values have increased.

Compared to baseline, statistically significant increase detected. For Average RNFL, Superior RNFL, Inferior RNFL, Rim Area values have increased. For Cup-to-Disc Ratios and Cup Volume values have decreased.

Figure 21-8 (continued). (B) Orange data points indicate possible RNFL loss, and red data points indicate likely RNFL loss.

Section V
Neuro-Ophthalmology

Section Editor
Wendy W. Lee, MD, MS

22

COMPUTED TOMOGRAPHY AND MAGNETIC RESONANCE IMAGING

Michelle W. Latting, MD
John W. Latting, MD
Sheikh Faheem, MD
Wendy W. Lee, MD, MS

Computed tomography (CT) and magnetic resonance imaging (MRI) are the most common radiologic studies used to visualize pathology of the orbit and visual pathway. Although plain film radiographs were once commonly utilized, the detail and anatomical information that can be gleaned from CT and MRI images are far superior. Plain film radiographs are still of value, however, particularly in the setting of trauma to exclude retained metallic foreign bodies prior to MRI.

CT imaging works by measuring the attenuation (absorption) of x-rays by structures located between the x-ray source and detector, whereas MRI measures the signal generated by radiofrequency excited hydrogen protons predominantly in fat and water. Because of the lack of freely-excited hydrogen protons in cortical bone and the relative paucity of marrow in facial bones, the bony structures of the orbit and skull are often best visualized with CT imaging. CT is therefore the study of choice in the setting of orbital fractures and to assess for bony erosion or destruction in the setting of space occupying tumors, malignancies, and other infiltrative processes.

One setting in which CT imaging may be inferior to MRI for visualizing bony detail is at the orbital apex. The presence of a high volume of dense bone at the orbital apex attenuates the x-ray beam to such an extent that too few x-rays reach the detector to create a quality image. For this reason, an MRI of the orbital apex may be superior to a CT. For example, crowding of the optic nerve at the orbital apex in the setting of thyroid eye disease may be better visualized with MRI than CT, although for most patients CT is adequate.

A CT window is a range of attenuation above which all attenuation values are assigned the same bright or white intensity, and below which all attenuation values are assigned the same dark or black intensity. Moving the window toward the lower range of attenuations allows for greater contrast between lower density tissues, such as fat and air, allowing soft tissue pathology to be better visualized. Moving the window toward the higher range of attenuation creates greater contrast

Gologorsky D, Rosen RB, eds.
Principles of Ocular Imaging (pp 201-212).
© 2021 Taylor & Francis Group.

between bone of varying densities. When viewing CT images one can manually adjust the window in a graded fashion, or select preset bone or soft tissue windows to best visualize the structures of interest. Orbital fractures are best visualized with a bone window, while the soft tissues of the orbit are best visualized with a soft tissue window.

A non-contrast CT scan is sufficient for the diagnosis of a variety of orbital pathology, including orbital fractures and thyroid eye disease. The administration of iodinated IV contrast media provides additional diagnostic information in the setting of vascular, inflammatory, infiltrative, and neoplastic processes, including intracranial extension. Inflammatory and neoplastic processes cause a breakdown in the blood-brain barrier allowing IV contrast material to pass into the surrounding tissues, resulting in contrast enhancement in the area of pathology.

Although some visualization of the orbits may be obtained with a CT of the head, a usual head CT is often displayed with larger 5 mm slices. The thinner 1 to 3 mm slices used for a dedicated orbital study provide greater resolution, albeit at the cost of decreased contrast.

A CT scan involves exposure to ionizing radiation, therefore the benefits of imaging must be weighed against the long term risks of tissue damage and potential malignancy. This is particularly true for pregnant women and children. CT contrast agents are relatively contraindicated in patients with renal failure (creatinine of 2.0 mg/dL or greater) and those with a prior anaphylactic reaction to iodinated contrast. Allergies to shellfish and topical iodine have historically been contraindications to iodinated contrast, but recent studies show a lack of correlation between these allergies and intravenous iodinated contrast reactions. However, not all hospitals' policies reflect this change in thought.

The physics of MRI is complex and beyond the scope of this reference. In general, MRI relies on the alignment of polarized atomic nuclei (usually hydrogen protons). When placed in a static magnetic field, the dipole electromagnetic moment created by the proton moving about the nucleus will align with the external magnetic field creating a resting state. Following excitation by a radiofrequency pulse or wave, at an energy absorbed by the proton in the hydrogen atom nucleus, these protons will move out of alignment with the magnetic field to an excited or higher energy state. In this higher energy state the excited protons rotate about the axis of the magnetic field like a spinning top that has been knocked off its axis of rotation. While the radiofrequency pulse is turned on the excited protons are pointing in the same direction. The sum of magnetic moments of the excited protons can be measured and creates an MRI signal. When the radiofrequency pulse is stopped, signal is lost in two major processes: signal is lost because protons return to their resting state (T1 relaxation) and signal is lost as protons fall out of alignment with each other because they rotate at different speeds (T2 relaxation or dephasing). In other words, T1 signal loss occurs because protons realign themselves with the external magnetic field, and T2 signal loss occurs because the sum of electromagnetic moments for the excited protons becomes more random and moves towards zero. The rates of T1 and T2 relaxation are determined by the properties of their atomic bonds. Fat, water, and proteins all have different T1 and T2 properties and these differences are exploited by each MRI sequence. The summation of the magnetic moments created by these excited protons induces a measurable current within an MRI coil placed around the imaged body part. A complex computer algorithm uses the information gathered to produce an image using a mathematical process called Fourier transformation.

Protons in water and fat within the human body are by far the main source of hydrogen protons in the body, and therefore contribute to the vast majority of signal used to create magnetic resonance images. In the face, soft tissues have a high water and fat content compared to bone, and therefore produce higher signal on MRI. This is why MRI is a great choice for imaging soft tissues in the face, but a poorer option for imaging bones.

T1-weighted images and T2-weighted images conceptually rely on the differences in the relaxation times of various molecules. For example, hydrogen protons in fat have a faster T1 relaxation time than hydrogen protons in water. Conceptually, it is easier to think of T1-weighted images as predominantly comprised of signal from molecules that have faster T1 relaxation times and T2 images as predominantly comprised of signal from molecules that have slower T1 relaxation times. This is a drastic oversimplification as it ignores T2 relaxation, and falsely suggests that there is a direct relationship between T1 and T2 properties. Nevertheless, this framework is good for a basic understanding. On T1-weighted images, tissues with high fat content (such as white matter) appear bright, while tissues with high water content (such as vitreous) appear dark. The opposite is true for T2-weighted images, in which tissues with high fat content appear dark and tissues with high water content appear bright.

Unless contraindicated, MRI studies of the orbit and brain should be ordered both with and without intravenous contrast. MRI imaging contrast is gadolinium based. Gadolinium creates contrast on MRI by shortening the relaxation time of protons in its immediate vicinity making them bright on T1-weighted images. It should be noted that the signal from fat is routinely suppressed on T2-weighted images and on many post-contrast, T1-weighted images to improve lesion conspicuity. For example, in the orbit, which contains significant fat, an enhancing lesion can be missed amidst the bright signal of the orbital fat on both the T2 and post-contrast, T1-weighted images. As such, studies of this region are routinely performed with fat suppression.

Allergic reactions to gadolinium occur much less frequently than reactions to CT contrast, and cross reactivity is uncommon. Therefore, a prior anaphylactic reaction to CT contrast is not a contraindication to gadolinium administration. Renal failure, however, is a contraindication to both CT and to many MRI contrast agents. As such, the appropriate gadolinium agent should be used cautiously in patients with a glomerular filtration rate less than 30 mL/min/1.73 m^2 to avoid the patient developing nephrogenic systemic fibrosis.

T2-weighted images allow for the visualization of inflammatory processes and other pathology associated with a relatively high water content (recall that on T2-weighted images water is bright). In acute optic neuritis, edema within the optic nerve can be visualized on T2-weighted imaging. If optic neuritis is suspected, an MRI of the brain should be ordered in addition to the orbital study in order to assess for demyelinating lesions. Fluid-attenuated inversion recovery (FLAIR) is a useful imaging sequence when evaluating for demyelinating lesions. FLAIR is conventionally performed with a T2-weighted technique and can be thought of as a T2-weighted image in which the signal from water (such as CSF and vitreous) is suppressed and will be dark (similar to that seen in T1-weighted images). Fluid associated with inflammatory processes, such as edema, will not be suppressed on FLAIR images and will be bright, allowing for better visualization of acute demyelinating lesions. It is important to note that gliosis will also be bright on T2-weighted images, including FLAIR. Therefore, in the setting of chronic demyelinating diseases, contrast enhancement is required to identify active lesions. In chronic demyelinating lesions the blood-brain barrier is restored and they will no longer enhance.

MRI is contraindicated in patients with metallic foreign bodies. In the setting of trauma or in those with a history of possible retained metallic foreign body, a plain film radiograph or CT study should be obtained to confirm the absence of metal prior to MRI. Most modern prostheses are made of non-ferromagnetic materials and are listed by the manufacturer as either "MRI Safe" or "MRI Conditional" for patients allowed to undergo MRI imaging. Most MRI facilities require patients to produce documentation verifying the MRI compatibility of their hardware prior to imaging. Gold and platinum eyelid weights, placed for lagophthalmos and modern orbito-facial hardware utilized in facial fracture repair, are typically listed by their manufacturers as either MRI safe or conditional. When in doubt, contact the manufacturer of the implant to obtain information regarding its safety in patients undergoing MRI.

CT and MRI can be used to perform dedicated studies of the arterial and venous system with angiography and venography, respectively. Common indications for CT angiography (CTA) or MR angiography (MRA) include evaluation for cerebral aneurysm (eg, in the setting of a third nerve palsy), arteriovenous malformation, dural or carotid cavernous fistula, or carotid disease such as dissection, stenosis, or occlusion. Although catheter angiography remains the gold standard for imaging many arterial lesions, CTA and MRA have dramatically reduced the use of catheter angiography due to the small but significant risk of severe complications associated with traditional catheter angiography. Both CTA and MRA are performed with intravenous contrast, with the exception of imaging cerebral arteries which can be done without IV contrast using time of flight (TOF) technique. However, IV contrast angiography of the intracranial arteries remains superior to TOF technique, and the use of one or the other is institution dependent. The decision of whether to order a CTA or MRA will depend on a number of factors, such as availability of the testing modality and institutional preference.

CT or MR Venography is most commonly ordered by the ophthalmologist to exclude the presence of dural venous sinus thrombosis in a patient with papilledema or other evidence of increased intracranial pressure. Although evidence of dural venous sinus thrombosis can sometimes be seen on non-contrast CT or MRI studies (eg, as absent flow void on T2-weighted MRI images, or as altered signal intensity in the area of thrombus on T1-weighted images), CT or MR Venography improves sensitivity for detecting the presence of thrombus.

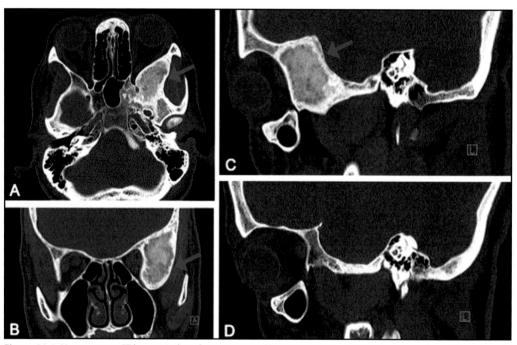

Figure 22-1. Non-contrast CT bone window demonstrating fibrous dysplasia of the left greater wing of the sphenoid (red arrows). (A) Axial slice. Notice the expansile, ground-glass appearance of the greater wing of the sphenoid, which contributes to the lateral orbital wall. (B) Coronal slice. Although not seen in this patient, expansion of the greater wing of the sphenoid can result in narrowing of the optic canal, superior orbital fissure, and inferior orbital fissure resulting in compressive optic neuropathy and other cranial neuropathies. (C) Sagittal slice demonstrating the affected left side. (D) Sagittal slice depicting the unaffected right side for comparison.

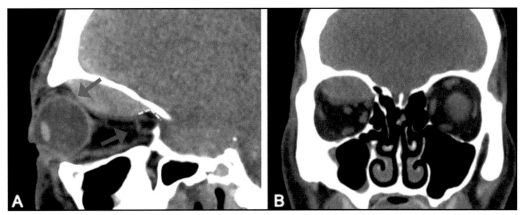

Figure 22-2. Non-contrast CT soft tissue window demonstrating subperiosteal abscess of the right orbit. (A) Sagittal slice demonstrating mass effect of the superior orbital lesion with inferior displacement of the optic nerve sheath complex (red arrow). The periosteum (blue arrow) is the thin linear density that is lifted off of the orbital roof by the underlying fluid collection. Notice the oblique margins of the lesion (yellow dashed lines) with the orbital roof, characteristic of a subperiosteal process. (B) Coronal slice demonstrating the extraconal soft tissue lesion within the superior right orbit. The posterior aspect of the globe is visible within the left orbit, but is not seen within the right orbit due to anterior displacement of the globe by the subperiosteal abscess causing right exophthalmos.

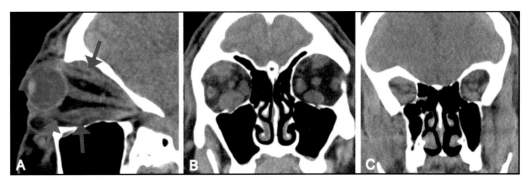

Figure 22-3. Non-contrast CT image soft tissue window demonstrating thyroid eye disease with bilateral extraocular muscle enlargement causing compressive optic neuropathy. (A) Sagittal slice demonstrating enlargement of the vertical rectus muscles (red arrows) with relative sparing of the muscle tendons (blue arrow). In contrast, other inflammatory and neoplastic processes involving the extraocular muscles tend to produce diffuse muscle enlargement involving both the muscle belly and tendinous attachments of the muscles to the globe. (B) Coronal slice through the anterior orbit demonstrating enlargement of the rectus muscles, right more than left orbit. Asymmetry of the extraocular muscles is best appreciated on coronal images. (C) Coronal slice through the posterior orbit. Notice the decreased ratio of fat to muscle near the orbital apex where compression of the optic nerve occurs.

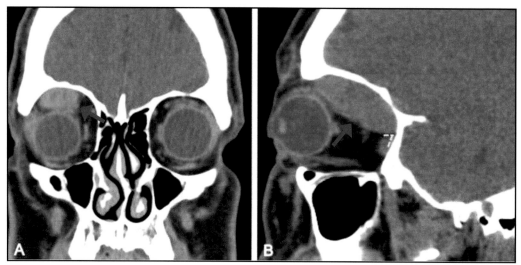

Figure 22-4. Non-contrast CT image soft tissue window demonstrating a schwannoma with-in the right superior orbit (red arrow). (A) Coronal slice. Notice the oval shape and relatively sharp margins. In general, a relatively well-circumscribed orbital mass is suggestive of a low-grade lesion. (B) Sagittal slice. The extraconal mass depicted here forms an acute angle (yellow dashed lines) with the orbital roof. Contrast this with the oblique angles of the subperiosteal collection in Figure 22-2.

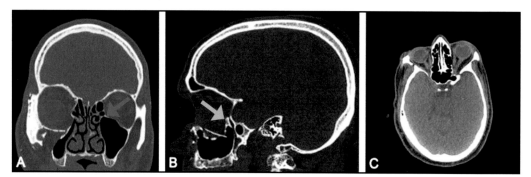

Figure 22-5. CT image demonstrating right orbital floor and lateral wall fractures with suboptimal reduction of the orbital floor fracture resulting in severe enophthalmos. Coronal and sagittal slices are best for viewing orbital floor fractures. At some institutions a CT of the head includes only thick axial slices in which small orbital floor fractures may be easily missed. Therefore, a dedicated CT study of the orbit is a necessity when orbital trauma is suspected. (A) Bone window coronal slice demonstrating a radiopaque plate spanning the fracture side over the lateral orbital rim and a radiopaque orbital floor implant, the medial aspect of which is inferiorly displaced and located within the maxillary sinus. The medial aspect of the implant should approximately correlate with the point at which the medial wall and floor of the contralateral orbit come together to form the orbital strut (blue arrow). Notice the increased volume of the right orbit due to the poorly positioned orbital floor implant. On the right, the globe is visualized in this section through the mid orbit due to the presence of severe enophthalmos. (B) Bone window sagittal slice demonstrating the posterior aspect of the orbital floor implant within the maxillary sinus. For optimal reduction of the fracture, the posterior aspect of the implant should rest at the posterior ledge of the maxillary sinus (green arrow). (C) Soft tissue window axial slice demonstrating enophthalmos of the right globe.

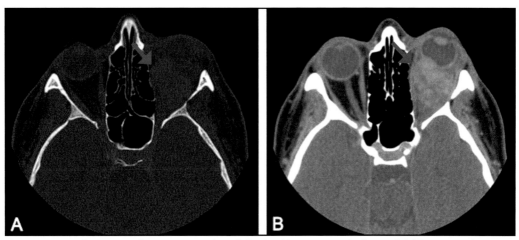

Figure 22-6. Axial CT images demonstrating a large left orbital hemangioma (red arrows). (A) Precontrast bone window. Although a large mass is visible within the left orbit, there is relatively poor soft tissue detail in this bone window. (B) Post-contrast soft tissue window. Notice the enhancement of the left orbital mass after contrast administration. Orbital hemangiomas are slow-flow lesions that slowly fill with contrast. Accordingly, enhancement patterns can vary depending on the phase of contrast imaging from peripheral-nodular enhancement, to heterogeneous enhancement (seen here), to homogeneous enhancement seen as the contrast equilibrates. Although not seen on these images, macroscopic fat and calcifications may be seen in orbital hemangiomas.

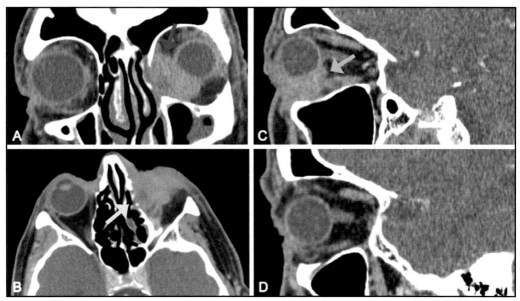

Figure 22-7. CT image soft tissue window demonstrating basal cell carcinoma of the left medial canthal region with extension into the orbit and involvement of the nasolacrimal sac. (A) Coronal slice demonstrating an infiltrative lesion (red arrow) within the left inferomedial orbit abutting the medial rectus and inferior rectus muscle. (B) Axial slice. Notice the destruction of bone along the medial orbital wall (yellow arrow). Slowly developing chronic processes, such as chronic sinusitis, cause thinning or expansion of adjacent bone. Bone loss and erosion are characteristic of aggressive processes such as infection and malignancy. (C) Sagittal slice through the affected left side. Compare the indistinct, poorly circumscribed margins (green arrow) of this aggressive process to the well-circumscribed margins of the low-grade schwannoma in Figure 22-4. (D) Sagittal slice demonstrating the contralateral unaffected side for comparison.

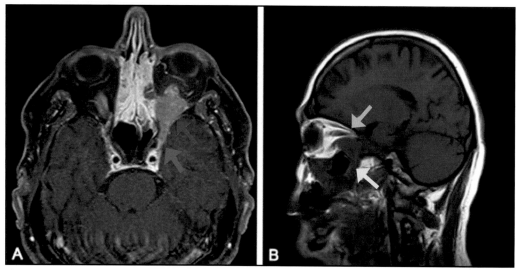

Figure 22-8. MRI image demonstrating diffuse large B-cell lymphoma involving the left orbital apex. (A) T1-weighted, post-contrast image with fat suppression, axial slice demonstrating an infiltrative lesion centered along the left orbital apex (red arrow) inseparable from the extraocular muscles with extension intracranially along the superior orbital fissure to the cavernous sinus (blue arrow). (B) T1-weighted image without fat suppression, sagittal slice demonstrating superior displacement of the optic nerve by the infiltrative lesion with compression of the optic nerve at the orbital apex (green arrow). The mass extends inferiorly, posterior to the maxillary sinus to involve the pterygopalatine fossa (yellow arrow).

Figure 22-9. Normal MRA. This image shows the anterior circulation including the intracranial carotid arteries (red arrows), bilateral middle cerebral arteries (yellow arrows), and parallel bilateral anterior cerebral arteries (blue arrows).

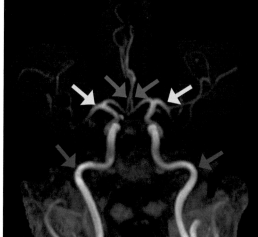

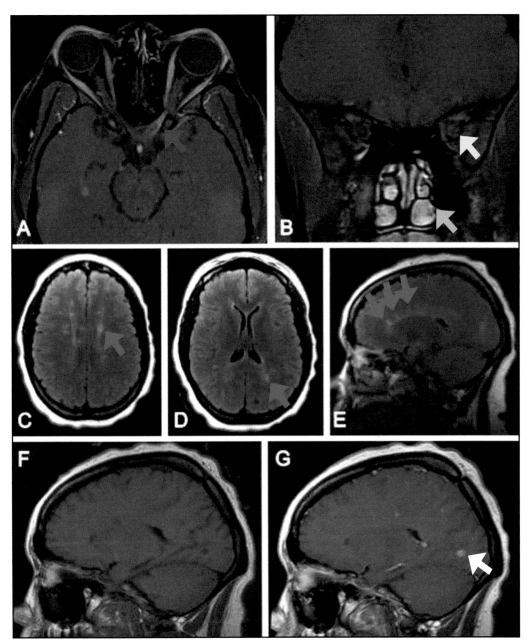

Figure 22-10. MRI images demonstrating left optic neuritis with periventricular demyelinating lesions suggestive of multiple sclerosis. (A) Axial post-contrast T1-weighted image with fat suppression demonstrating enhancement of the intracanalicular portion of the left optic nerve (red arrow). Enhancement is an important finding in active optic neuritis and is best seen on axial images. In contrast, coronal images are best for visualizing enlargement, or asymmetry of the optic nerve, seen with mass lesions of the optic nerve or nerve sheath. (B) Coronal post-contrast, T1-weighted image with fat suppression demonstrating subtle enhancement of the left optic nerve at the orbital apex (yellow arrow). Notice the avid enhancement of the nasal mucosa (green arrow), a characteristic finding on a post-contrast MRI image that distinguishes it from pre-contrast images. (C) Axial T2 FLAIR images show periventricular white matter involvement (blue arrow) characteristic of multiple sclerosis. (D) The white matter lesions of multiple sclerosis are best viewed on T2-weighted images. (E) Sagittal T2 FLAIR image, again demonstrating periventricular white matter involvement (blue arrows). This image demonstrates the characteristic appearance of "Dawson's fingers." Multiple sclerosis plaques typically extend retrograde from the periventricular regions along the subependymal and deep medullary veins, creating "finger-like" projections. This finding is best viewed on sagittal FLAIR images and distinguishes multiple sclerosis from white matter changes seen with chronic microvascular disease.

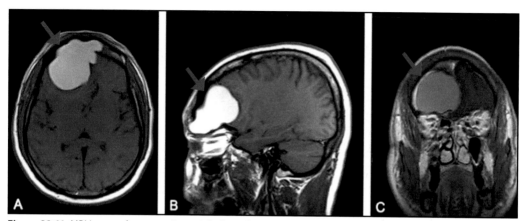

Figure 22-11. MRI images demonstrating a right frontal sinus mucocele (red arrows). The mucocele fills and expands the entire right frontal sinus causing mass effect on the surrounding structures. This process does not invade or destroy the bony sinus walls, which are thin and difficult to see. (A) Axial and (B) sagittal precontrast T1-weighted images demonstrate mass effect on the right frontal lobe and right orbital structures. The mucocele is intrinsically T1 hyperintense (bright) due to proteinaceous debris. (C) Coronal post-contrast T1-weighted image. Notice the brain parenchyma and mucocele are slightly darker in this image, though all of the images are T1 weighted. Signal intensity is relative in MRI. In images A and B, the mucocele was one of the brightest structures on the image. However, it is signal-poor relative to the signal-rich enhancing sinus mucosa in image C, and gets pushed down the display intensity scale.

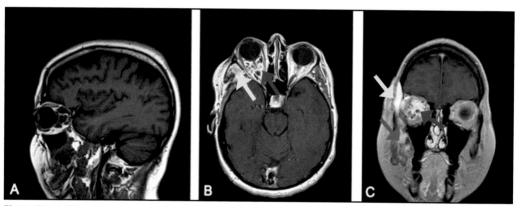

Figure 22-12. MRI images demonstrating a venous malformation involving the right orbit (red arrows), temporal fossa (yellow arrows), and masticator space (blue arrow). (A) Sagittal precontrast T1-weighted image. Notice the "serpiginous" T1 hypointense signal within the right orbit. (B) Axial and (C) coronal post-contrast T1 images show enhancement of the lesion and relative proptosis of the right globe.

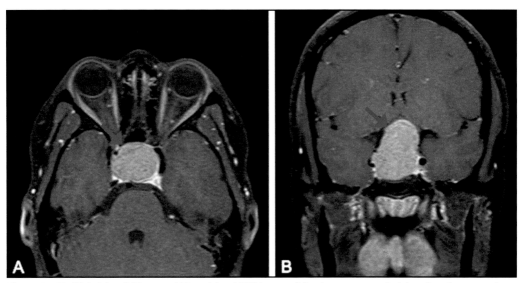

Figure 22-13. (A) Axial and (B) coronal T1-weighted MRI images following contrast administration demonstrating a pituitary macroadenoma (red arrow). The distinction between microadenoma and macroadenoma is made by size, with the threshold being 1 cm. The optic chiasm is compressed by the adenoma and is not visualized.

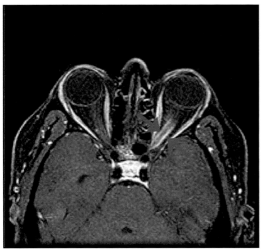

Figure 22-14. Axial T1-weighted MRI image following contrast administration demonstrating enhancement of the optic nerve sheath (red arrows) consistent with optic nerve sheath meningioma. Notice the characteristic "tram track" appearance which is caused by growth of the tumor along the meninges surrounding the optic nerve.

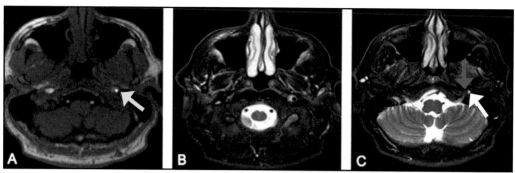

Figure 22-15. Left carotid artery dissection at the entry to the carotid canal in a patient with ipsilateral Horner's syndrome. MRI image, T1-weighted (A) pre-contrast and (B) post-contrast axial slices. Normal blood flow is typically bright on T1-weighted images and dark on T2-weighted images. Due to narrowing of the vessel lumen by the dissection, the bright signal corresponding to intraluminal blood flow on the precontrast T1-weighted image (A, yellow arrow) and the dark signal corresponding to intraluminal blood flow on the T2-weighted image (C, blue arrow) is reduced in size compared to the contralateral side. (C) MRI image, T2-weighted axial slice. Notice that the dark signal corresponding to intraluminal blood flow on the T2-weighted image (blue arrow) is reduced in size compared to the contralateral side. The T2 hyperintense signal within the vessel wall (white arrow) represents loss of the normal "flow void" due to stagnant blood within the dissection. (D) MRA three-dimensional reconstruction demonstrating an intraluminal filling defect (red arrow) caused by the dissection.

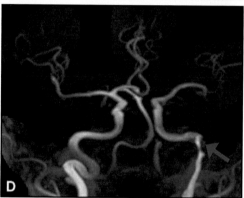

Bibliography

Chapter 1 External Photography

American Society of Ophthalmic Plastic and Reconstructive Surgery. White paper on functional blepharoplasty, blepharoptosis, and brow ptosis repair. American Society of Ophthalmic Plastic and Reconstructive Surgery. https://www.asoprs.org/assets/docs/1%20-%20FINAL%20ASOPRS%20White%20Paper%20January%202015.pdf. Published January 2015.

Jakowenko J. Clinical photography. *J Telemed Telecar*e. 2009;15(1):7-22. doi: 10.1258/jtt.2008.008006.

Mukherjee B, Nair AG. Principles and practice of external digital photography in ophthalmology. *Indian J Ophthalmol*. 2012;60(2):119-125. doi: 10.4103/0301-4738.94053.

Nayler JR. Clinical photography: a guide for the clinician. *J Postgrad Med*. 2003;Jul-Sep;49(3):256-262.

Persichetti P, Simone P, Langella M, Marangi GF, Carusi C. Digital photography in plastic surgery: how to achieve reasonable standardization outside a photographic studio. *Aesthetic Plast Surg*. 2007;31(2):194-200. doi: 10.1007/s00266-006-0125-5

Chapter 2 Ptosis Visual Fields

Alniemi ST, Pang NK, Woog JJ, Bradley EA. Comparison of automated and manual perimetry in patients with blepharoptosis. *Ophthalmic Plast Reconstr Surg*. 2013;29(5):361-363. doi: 10.1097/IOP.0b013e31829a7288

American Society of Ophthalmic Plastic and Reconstructive Surgery. White paper on functional blepharoplasty, blepharoptosis, and brow ptosis repair. American Society of Ophthalmic Plastic and Reconstructive Surgery. https://www.asoprs.org/assets/docs/1%20-%20FINAL%20ASOPRS%20White%20Paper%20January%202015.pdf. Published January 2015.

Ho SF, Morawski A, Sampath R, Burns J. Modified visual field test for ptosis surgery (Leicester Peripheral Field Test). *Eye (Lond)*. 201;25(3):365-369. doi: 10.1038/eye.2010.210

Gologorsky D, Rosen RB, eds.
Principles of Ocular Imaging (pp 213-222).
© 2021 Taylor & Francis Group.

Meyer DR, Stern JH, Jarvis JM, Lininger LL. Evaluating the visual field effects of blepharoptosis using automated static perimetry. *Ophthalmology.* 1993;100(5):651-659. doi: 10.1016/s0161-6420(93)31593-9

Wong SH, Plant GT. How to interpret visual fields. *Pract Neurol.* 2015;15(5):374-381. doi:10.1136/practneurol-2015-001155

CHAPTER 3 SLIT LAMP PHOTOGRAPHY

Ding J. How to use a slit lamp. American Academy of Ophthalmology. www.aao.org/young-ophthalmologists/yo-info/article/how-to-use-slit-lamp. Published May 24, 2016.

Flaherty S. Slit-lamp photography: the smart way. American Academy of Ophthalmology. www.aao.org/eyenet/article/slit-lamp-photography. Published November 2017.

Gilman J. Slit lamp biomicrography. Ophthalmic Photographers' Society. www.opsweb.org/page/slitbiomicrography.

Lowe R. Clinical slit lamp photography—an update. *Clin Exp Optom.* 1991;74(4):125-129.

Slit Lamp Imaging Guide. Haag Streit International. https://innovamed.com/sites/default/files/downloads/BX900-Photo-guide.pdf

CHAPTER 4 ORBITAL ULTRASONOGRAPHY

Dick AD, Nangia V, Atta H. Standardised echography in the differential diagnosis of extraocular muscle enlargement. *Eye (Lond).* 1992;6(Pt 6):610-617. doi: 10.1038/eye.1992.132

Kendall CJ, Prager TC, Cheng H, Gombos D, Tang RA, Schiffman JS. Diagnostic ophthalmic ultrasound for radiologists. *Neuroimaging Clin N Am.* 2015;25(3):327-365. doi: 10.1016/j.nic.2015.05.001

Mundt GH Jr, Hughes WF Jr. Ultrasonics in ocular diagnosis. *Am J Ophthalmol.* 2018;189:xxviii-xxxvi. doi: 10.1016/j.ajo.2018.02.017

Ossoinig KC. Standardized echography: basic principles, clinical applications, and results. *Int Ophthalmol Clin.* 1979;19(4):127-210.

Smoker WR, Gentry LR, Yee NK, Reede DL, Nerad JA. Vascular lesions of the orbit: more than meets the eye. *Radiographics.* 2008;28(1):185-204; quiz 325. doi: 10.1148/rg.281075040

Williamson TH, Harris A. Color Doppler ultrasound imaging of the eye and orbit. *Surv Ophthalmol.* 1996;40(4):255-267. doi: 10.1016/s0039-6257(96)82001-7

CHAPTER 5 CORNEAL TOPOGRAPHY

Anderson D, Kojima R. Topography: a clinical pearl. *Optom Manag.* 2007;42(2):35.

Brody J, Waller S, Wagoner M. Corneal topography: history, technique, and clinical uses. *Int Ophthalmol Clin.* 1994;34(3):197-207. doi: 10.1097/00004397-199403430-00018

Examination techniques for the external eye and cornea. In: Basic and Clinical Science Course (BCSC) Section 8: External Disease and Cornea. San Francisco, CA: American Academy of Ophthalmology; 2014:24-30.

Greenwald MF, Scruggs BA, Vislisel JM, Greiner MA. Corneal imaging: an introduction. EyeRounds.org. eyerounds.org/tutorials/corneal-imaging/index.htm. Published October 19, 2016.

Oliveira CM, Ribeiro C, Franco S. Corneal imaging with slit-scanning and Scheimpflug imaging techniques. *Clin Exp Optom.* 2011;94(1):33-42. doi: 10.1111/j.1444-0938.2010.00509.x

Chapter 6 Confocal Microscopy

Chiou AG, Kaufman SC, Kaufman HE, Beuerman RW. Clinical corneal confocal microscopy. *Surv Ophthalmol.* 2006;51(5):482-500. doi: 10.1016/j.survophthal.2006.06.010

Confocal microscopy. American Academy of Ophthalmology. www.aao.org/focalpointssnip petdetail.aspx?id=646c324e-cc30-48db-8896-07a24b5fd28a.

Erie JC, Mclaren JW, Patel SV. Confocal microscopy in ophthalmology. *Am J Ophthalmol.* 2009;148(5):639-646. doi: 10.1016/j.ajo.2009.06.022

Kaufman SC, Musch DC, Belin MW, et al. Confocal microscopy: a report by the American Academy of Ophthalmology. *Ophthalmology.* 2004;111(2):396-406. doi: 10.1016/j.ophtha.2003.12.002

Tavakoli M, Hossain P, Malik RA. Clinical applications of corneal confocal microscopy. *Clin Ophthalmol.* 2008;2(2):435-445. doi: 10.2147/opth.s1490

Chapter 7 Anterior Segment Optical Coherence Tomography

Han SB, Liu YC, Noriega KM, Mehta JS. Applications of anterior segment optical coherence tomography in cornea and ocular surface diseases. *J Ophthalmol.* 2016;2016:4971572. doi: 10.1155/2016/4971572

Karp CL. Evolving technologies for lid and ocular surface neoplasias: is optical biopsy a reality? *JAMA Ophthalmol.* 2017;135(8):852-853. doi: 10.1001/jamaophthalmol.2017.2009

Shousha MA, Karp CL, Canto AP, et al. Diagnosis of ocular surface lesions using ultra-high-resolution optical coherence tomography. *Ophthalmology.* 2013;120(5):883-891. doi: 10.1016/j.ophtha.2012.10.025

Thomas BJ, Galor A, Nanji AA, et al. Ultra high-resolution anterior segment optical coherence tomography in the diagnosis and management of ocular surface squamous neoplasia. *Ocul Surf.* 2014;12(1):46-58. doi: 10.1016/j.jtos.2013.11.001

Wang J, Abou Shousha M, Perez VL, et al. Ultra-high resolution optical coherence tomography for imaging the anterior segment of the eye. *Ophthalmic Surg Lasers Imaging.* 2011;42 (Suppl):S15-S27. doi: 10.3928/15428877-20110627-02

Chapter 8 Ultrasound Biomicroscopy

Dada T, Gadia R, Sharma A, et al. Ultrasound biomicroscopy in glaucoma. *Surv Ophthalmol.* 2011; 56(5):433-450. doi: 10.1016/j.survophthal.2011.04.004

He M, Wang D, Jiang Y. Overview of ultrasound biomicroscopy. *J Curr Glaucoma Pract.* 2012;6(1):25-53. doi: 10.5005/jp-journals-10008-1105

Ishikawa H. Anterior segment imaging for glaucoma: OCT or UBM? *Br J Ophthalmol.* 2007;91(11):1420-1421. doi: 10.1136/bjo.2007.121038

Pavlin CJ, Harasiewicz K, Sherar MD, Foster FS. Clinical use of ultrasound biomicroscopy. *Ophthalmology.* 1991;98(3):287-295. doi: 10.1016/s0161-6420(91)32298-x

Pavlin CJ, Sherar MD, Foster FS. Subsurface ultrasound microscopic imaging of the intact eye. *Ophthalmology.* 1990;97(2):244-250. doi: 10.1016/s0161-6420(90)32598-8

CHAPTER 9 BIOMETRY FOR INTRAOCULAR LENS CALCULATIONS

Byrne SF. *A-Scan Axial Length Measurements: A Handbook for IOL Calculations*. New York, NY: Grove Park Publishers; 1995.

Emerson JH, Tompkins K. IOLMaster: A Practical Operation Guide. Carl Zeiss Meditec, Inc. www.doctor-hill.com/physicians/docs/IOLMaster_Practical_Operation_Guide.pdf

Friedman NJ. Instrument Basics Part I: Biometry. Ophthalmology Web. www.ophthal mologyweb.com/Tech-Spotlights/26492-Instrument-Basics-Part-I-Biometry/. Published: October 2, 2008.

Sahin A, Hamrah P. Clinically relevant biometry. *Curr Opin Ophthalmol*. 2012;23(1):47-53. doi: 10.1097/ICU.0b013e32834cd63e

Waldron RG, Aaberg TM Jr. A-Scan Biometry. Medscape. emedicine.medscape.com/article /1228447-overview. Updated: Apr 20, 2016.

CHAPTER 10 FUNDUS PHOTOGRAPHY

Fundus Photography Overview. Ophthalmic Photographers' Society. www.opsweb.org. Retrieved 2019-10-31.

Haddock LJ, Kim DY, Mukai S. Simple, inexpensive technique for high-quality smartphone fundus photography in human and animal eyes. *J Ophthalmol*. 2013;518479.

Hansell P, Beeson EJG. Retinal photography in colour. *Br J Ophthalmol*. 1953;37:65-69. doi: 10.1136/bjo.37.2.65

Jackman WT, Webster JD. On photographing the retina of the living human eye. *The Philadelphia Photographer*. 1886;23:340 341.

Nazari Khanamiri H, Nakatsuka A, El-Annan J. Smartphone fundus photography. *J Vis Exp*. 2017;(125). doi: 10.3791/55958

Panwar N, Huang P, Lee J, et al. Fundus photography in the 21st century—a review of recent technological advances and their implications for worldwide healthcare. *Telemed J E Health*. 2016;22(3):198-208. doi: 10.1089/tmj.2015.0068

CHAPTER 11 FLUORESCEIN ANGIOGRAPHY

Bennett TJ. Descriptive interpretation. Ophthalmic Photographers' Society. https://www .opsweb.org/page/Fainterpretation.

Gass JDM, Sever RJ, Sparks D, Goren J. A combined technique of fluorescein fun-doscopy and angiography of the eye. *Arch Ophthalmol*. 1967;78:455-461. doi: 10.1001/ archopht.1967.00980030457009

Novotny HR, Alvis DL. A method of photographing fluorescence in circulating blood in the human retina. *Circulation*. 1961;24:82-86.

Rabb MF, Burton TC, Schatz H, Yannuzzi LA. Fluorescein angiography of the fundus: a schematic approach to interpretation. *Surv Ophthalmol*. 1978;22:387-403. doi: 10.1016/0039-6257(78)90134-0

Schatz H, Burton TC, Yanuzzi LA, Rabb MF. *Interpretation of fundus fluorescein angiography*. St. Louis, MO; Mosby-Year Book :1978.

Yannuzzi LA, Rohrer, MA, Tindel LJ, et al. Fluorescein angiography complication survey. *Ophthalmology*. 1986;93:611-617. doi: 10.1016/s0161-6420(86)33697-2

Young CW. Interpretation of fundus fluorescein angiography. *Arch Ophthalmol*. 1979;97:564-565. doi:10.1001/archopht.1979.01020010300028

CHAPTER 12 INDOCYANINE GREEN ANGIOGRAPHY

Hayashi K, Hasegawa Y, Tazawa Y, De Laey JJ. Clinical application of indocyanine green angiography to choroidal neovascularization. *Jpn J Ophthalmol*. 1989;33(1):57-65.

Hochheimer BF. Angiography of the retina with indocyanine green. *Arch Ophthalmol*. 1971;86:564-565.

Miller KR. Indocyanine green angiography. Ophthalmic Photographers' Society. https://www.opsweb.org/page/ICG

Owens SL. Indocyanine green angiography. *Br J Ophthalmol*. 1996;80(3):263-266. doi: 10.1136/bjo.80.3.263

Patz A, Flower RW, Klein MI, et al, Clinical applications of indocyanine green angiography. *Doc Ophthalmol Proc Sev*. 1976;9:245-251.

Stanga PE, Lim JL, Hamilton P. Indocyanine green angiography in chorioretinal diseases: an evidence-based update. *Ophthalmology*. 2003;110:15-21. doi: 10.1016/s0161-6420(02)01563-4

Yannuzzi LA. Indocyanine green angiography: a perspective on use in the clinical setting. *Am J Ophthalmol*. 2011;151(5):745-751.e1. doi: 10.1016/j.ajo.2011.01.043

Yannuzzi LA, Slakter JS, Sorenson JA, Guyer DR, Orlock DA. Digital indocyanine green videoangiography and choroidal neovascularization. *Retina*. 1992;12(3):191-223.

CHAPTER 13 FUNDUS AUTOFLUORESCENCE

Boon C, Klevering B, Keunen J, Hoyng CB, Theelen T. Fundus autofluorescence imaging of retinal dystrophies. *Vision Res*. 2008:48(26):2569-2577. doi: 10.1016/j.visres.2008.01.010

Durrani K, Foster CS. Fundus autofluorescence imaging in posterior uveitis. *Semin Ophthalmol*. 2012;27(5-6):228-235. doi: 10.3109/08820538.2012.711414

Holz FG, Schmitz-Valckenberg S, Spaide RF, Bird AC. *Atlas of Fundus Autofluorescence Imaging*. Berlin, Germany: Springer-Verlag; 2007.

Meleth AD, Sen HN. Use of fundus autofluorescence in the diagnosis and management of uveitis. *Int Ophthalmol Clin*. 2012;52(4):45-54. doi: 10.1097/IIO.0b013e3182662ee9

Yung M, Klufas MA, Sarraf D. Clinical applications of fundus autofluorescence in retinal disease. *Int J Retina Vitreous*. 2016;2-12. doi: 10.1186/s40942-016-0035-x

CHAPTER 14 OPTICAL COHERENCE TOMOGRAPHY IN RETINA

Adhi M, Duker JS. Optical coherence tomography—current and future applications. *Curr Opin Ophthalmol*. 2013;24(3):213-221. doi: 10.1097/ICU.0b013e32835f8bf8

Gabriele ML, Wollstein G, Ishikawa H, et al. Optical coherence tomography: history, current status, and laboratory work. *Invest Ophthalmol Vis Sci*. 2011;52(5):2425-2436. doi: 10.1167/iovs.10-6312

Huang D, Swanson EA, Lin CP, et al. Optical coherence tomography. *Science.* 1991;254(5035): 1178-1181. doi: 10.1126/science.1957169

Ishikawa H, Stein DM, Wollstein G, Beaton S, Fujimoto JG, Schuman JS. Macular segmentation with optical coherence tomography. *Invest Ophthalmol Vis Sci.* 2005;46:2012-2017. doi: 10.1167/iovs.04-0335

Leitgeb R, Hitzenberger C, Fercher A. Performance of fourier domain vs. time domain optical coherence tomography. *Opt Express.* 2003;11:889-894. doi: 10.1364/oe.11.000889

Margolis R, Spaide RF. A pilot study of enhanced depth imaging optical coherence tomography of the choroid in normal eyes. *Am J Ophthalmol.* 2009;147(5):811-815. doi: 10.1016/j.ajo.2008.12.008

Mrejen S, Spaide RF. Optical coherence tomography: imaging of the choroid and beyond. *Surv Ophthalmol.* 2013;58(5):387-429. doi: 10.1016/j.survophthal.2012.12.001

Spaide RF, Koizumi H, Pozzoni MC. Enhanced depth imaging spectral-domain optical coherence tomography. *Am J Ophthalmol.* 2008;146:496-500. doi: 10.1016/j.ajo.2008.05.032.

Strong J. Optical coherence tomography (OCT). Ophthalmic Photographers' Society. https://www.opsweb.org/page/RetinalOCT

Sull AC, Vuong LN, Price LL, et al. Comparison of spectral/Fourier domain optical coherence tomography instruments for assessment of normal macular thickness. *Retina.* 2010;30(2):235-245. doi: 10.1097/IAE.0b013e3181bd2c3b

CHAPTER 15 OPTICAL COHERENCE TOMOGRAPHY ANGIOGRAPHY

Agemy SA, Scripsema NK, Shah CM, et al. Retinal vascular perfusion density mapping using optical coherence tomography angiography in normal and diabetic retinopathy patients. *Retina.* 2015;35:2353-2363. doi: 10.1097/IAE.0000000000000862

Huang D, Swanson EA, Lin CP, et al. Optical coherence tomography. *Science.* 1991;22;254:1178-1181. doi: 10.1126/science.1957169

Kashani AH, Chen CL, Gahm JK, et al. Optical coherence tomography angiography: a comprehensive review of current methods and clinical applications. *Prog Retin Eye Res.* 2017;60:66-100. doi: 10.1016/j.preteyeres.2017.07.002

Nehemy MB, Brocchi DN, Veloso CE. Optical coherence tomography imaging of quiescent choroidal neovascularization in age-related macular degeneration. *Ophthalmic Surg Lasers Imaging Retina.* 2015;46:1056-1057. doi: 10.3928/23258160-20151027-13

Sambhav K, Grover S, Chalam KV. The application of optical coherence tomography angiography in retinal diseases. *Surv Ophthalmol.* 2017;62(6):838-866. doi: 10.1016/j.survophthal.2017.05.006

Spaide RF, Fujimoto JG, Waheed NK, Sadda SR, Staurenghi G. Optical coherence tomography angiography. *Prog Retin Eye Res.* 2018;64:1-55. doi: 10.1016/j.preteyeres.2017.11.003

Wu CY, Garcia P, Rosen RB. Multimodal imaging of progressive outer retinal necrosis. *Ophthalmol Retina.* 2019;3(1):41. doi: 10.1016/j.oret.2018.10.001

CHAPTER 16 ADAPTIVE OPTICS

Burns SA, Elsner AE, Sapoznik KA, Warner Rl, Gast TJ. Adaptive optics imaging of the human retina. *Prog Retin Eye Res.* 2018; 26 Aug 2018, 68:1-30. doi: 10.1016/j.preteyeres.2018.08.002

Chui TYP, Pinhas A, Gan A, et al. Longitudinal imaging of microvascular remodeling in proliferative diabetic retinopathy using adaptive optics scanning light ophthalmoscopy. *Ophthalmic Physiol Opt.* 2016;36(3):290-302. doi: 10.1111/opo

Dreher AW, Bille JF, Weinreb RN. Active optical depth resolution improvement of the laser tomographic scanner. *Appl Optic.* 1989;28(4):804-808. doi: 10.1364/AO.28.000804

Dubis AM, Cooper RF, Aboshiha J, et al. Genotype-dependent variability in residual cone structure in achromatopsia: toward developing metrics for assessing cone health. *Invest Ophthalmol Vis Sci.* 2014;55(11):7303-7311. doi: 10.1167/iovs.14-14225

Dubow M, Pinhas A, Shah N, et al. Classification of human retinal microaneurysms using adaptive optics scanning light ophthalmoscope fluorescein angiography. *Invest Ophthalmol Vis Sci.* 2014;55:1299-1309. doi: 10.1167/iovs.13-13122

Dubra A, Sulai Y, Norris JL, et al. Noninvasive imaging of the human rod photoreceptor mosaic using a confocal adaptive optics scanning ophthalmoscope. *Biomed Opt Express.* 2011;2(7):1864-1876. doi: 10.1364/BOE.2.001864

Flatter JA, Cooper RF, Dubow MJ, et al. Outer retinal structure after closed-globe blunt ocular trauma. *Retina.* 2014;34(10):2133-2146. doi: 10.1097/IAE.0000000000000169

Genead MA, Fishman GA, Rha J, et al. Photoreceptor structure and function in patients with congenital achromatopsia. *Invest Ophthalmol Vis Sci.* 2011;52:7298-7308. doi: 10.1167/iovs.11-7762

Hood DC, Chen MF, Lee D, et al. Confocal adaptive optics imaging of peripapillary nerve fiber bundles: implications for glaucomatous damage seen on circumpapillary OCT scans. *Transl Vis Sci Technol.* 2015;4(2):12. doi: 10.1167/tvst.4.2.12

Huang G, Gast TJ, Burns SA. In vivo adaptive optics imaging of the temporal raphe and its relationship to the optic disc and fovea in the human retina. *Invest Ophthalmol Vis Sci.* 2014;55(9):5952-5961. doi: 10.1167/iovs.14-14893

Liang J, Williams DR, Miller DT. Supernormal vision and high-resolution retinal imaging through adaptive optics. *J Opt Soc Am A Opt Image Sci Vis.* 1997;14(11):2884-2892. doi: 10.1364/josaa.14.002884

Pinhas A, Dubow M, Shah N, et al. Fellow eye changes in patients with nonischemic central retinal vein occlusion: assessment of perfused foveal microvascular density and identification of nonperfused capillaries. *Retina 2015*;35:2028-2036

Plesch A, Klingbeil U, Bille J. Digital laser scanning fundus camera. *Appl Optic.* 1987;26:1480-1586. doi: 10.1364/AO.26.001480

Roorda A, Duncan JL. Adaptive optics ophthalmoscopy. *Annu Rev Vis Sci.* 2015;1:19-50. doi: 10.1146/annurev-vision-082114-035357

Roorda A, Williams DR. The arrangement of the three cone classes in the living human eye. *Nature.* 1999;397(6719):520-522. doi: 10.1038/17383

Scoles D, Sulai YN, Dubra A. In vivo dark-field imaging of the retinal pigment epithelium cell mosaic. *Biomed Optic Express.* 2013;4(9):1710-1723. doi: 10.1364/BOE.4.001710

Wu CY, Jansen ME, Andrade J, et al. Acute solar retinopathy imaged with adaptive optics, optical coherence tomography angiography, and en face optical coherence tomography. *JAMA Ophthalmol.* 2018;136(1):82-85. doi: 10.1001/jamaophthalmol.2017.5517

Yanoga F, Gentile RC, Chui TYP, et al. Sildenafil citrate induced retinal toxicity—eletroretinogram, optical coherence tomography, and adaptive optics findings. *Retin Cases Brief Rep.* 2018;12(Suppl 1):S33-S40. doi: 10.1097/ICB.0000000000000708

CHAPTER 17 MICROPERIMETRY

Acton JH, Greenstein VC. Fundus-driven perimetry (microperimetry) compared to conventional static automated perimetry: similarities, differences, and clinical applications. *Can J Ophthalmol*. 2013;48:358-363. doi: 10.1016/j.jcjo.2013.03.021

Cassels NK, Wild JM, Margrain TH, Chong V, Acton JH. The use of microperimetry in assessing visual function in age-related macular degeneration. *Surv Ophthalmol*. 2018;63(1):40-55. doi: 10.1016/j.survophthal.2017.05.007

Hanout M, Horan N, Do DV. Introduction to microperimetry and its use in analysis of geographic atrophy in age-related macular degeneration. *Curr Opinion Ophthalmol*. 2015;26(3):149-156.

Laishram M, Srikanth K, Rajalakshmi AR, Nagarajan S, Ezhumalai G. Microperimetry—a new tool for assessing retinal sensitivity in macular diseases. *J Clin Diagn Res*. 2017;11(7):NC08-NC11. doi: 10.7860/JCDR/2017/25799.10213

Markowitz SN, Reyes SV. Microperimetry and clinical practice: an evidence-based review. *Can J Ophthalmol*. 2013;48(5):350-357. doi: 10.1016/j.jcjo.2012.03.004

CHAPTER 18 RETINAL ULTRASONOGRAPHY

Coleman DJ, Silverman RH, Chabi A, et al. High resolution ultrasonic imaging of the posterior segment. *Ophthalmology*. 2004;111(7):1344-1351. doi: 10.1016/j.ophtha.2003.10.029

De La Hoz Polo M, Torramilans Lluís A, Pozuelo Segura O, et al. Ocular ultrasonography focused on the posterior eye segment: what radiologists should know. *Insights Imaging*. 2016;7(3):351-364. doi: 10.1007/s13244-016-0471-z

Hewick SA, Fairhead AC, Culy JC, Atta HR. A comparison of 10 MHz and 20 MHz ultrasound probes in imaging the eye and orbit. *Br J Ophthalmol*. 2004;88(4):551-555. doi: 10.1136/bjo.2003.028126

Mundt G Jr, Hughes W Jr. Ultrasonics in ocular diagnosis. *Am J Ophthalmol*. 1956;41(3):488-498.

Oksala A, Lehtinen A. Diagnostic value of ultrasonics in ophthalmology. *Ophthalmologica*. 1957;134(6):387-395. doi: 10.1159/000303246

Silverman RH. Focused ultrasound in ophthalmology. *Clin Ophthalmol*. 2016;10:1865–75. doi:10.2147/OPTH.S99535 https://ophthalmicedge.org/physician/course/?Imaging/Ultrasound/18

CHAPTER 19 ELECTROPHYSIOLOGY OF VISION

Constable PA, Bach M, Frishman LJ, Jeffrey BG, Robson AG. ISCEV standard for clinical electro-oculography. *Doc Ophthalmol*. 2017;134:1-9. doi: 10.1007/s10633-017-9573-2

Hood DC, Bach M, Brigell M, et al. ISCEV standard for clinical multifocal electroretinography. *Doc Ophthalmol*. 2012;124(1):1-13. doi: 10.1007/s10633-011-9296-8

McCulloch DL, Marmor MF, Brigell MG, et al. ISCEV standard for full field clinical electroretinography. *Doc Ophthalmol*. 2015;130(1):1-12. doi: 10.1007/s10633-014-9473-7

Odom JV, Bach M, Brigell M, et al. ISCEV standard for for clinical visually evoked potential. *Doc Ophthalmol*. 2016;133(1):1-9. doi: 10.1007/s10633-016-9553-y

Robson A, Nilsson J, Li S, et al. ISCEV guide to visual electrodiagnostic procedure. *Doc Ophthalmol*. 2018;136(1):1-26. doi: 10.1007/s10633-017-9621-y

CHAPTER 20 VISUAL FIELDS IN GLAUCOMA

Budenz DL, Rhee P, Feuer WJ, McSoley J, Johnson CA, Anderson DR. Comparison of glaucomatous visual field defects using standard full threshold and Swedish interactive threshold algorithms. *Arch Ophthalmol.* 2002;120(9):1136-1141. doi: 10.1001/archopht.120.9.1136

Chakravarti T. Assessing precision of Hodapp-Parrish-Anderson criteria for staging early glaucomatous damage in an ocular hypertension cohort: a retrospective study. *Asia Pac J Ophthalmol (Phila).* 2017;6(1):21-27. doi: 10.1097/APO.0000000000000201

Chen Chang T, Ramulu P, Hodapp E. *Clinical Decisions in Glaucoma.* Miami, FL: Bascom Palmer Eye Institute; 2016.

Keltner JL, Johnson CA, Quigg JM, Cello KE, Kass MA, Gordon MO. Confirmation of visual field abnormalities in the Ocular Hypertension Treatment Study. Ocular Hypertension Treatment Study Group. *Arch Ophthalmol.* 2000;118(9):1187-1194. doi: 10.1001/archopht.118.9.1187

Mills RP, Budenz DL, Lee PP, et al. Categorizing the stage of glaucoma from pre-diagnosis to end-stage disease. *Am J Ophthalmol.* 2006;141(1):24-30. doi: 10.1016/j.ajo.2005.07.044

CHAPTER 21 OPTICAL COHERENCE TOMOGRAPHY IN GLAUCOMA

Chen TC, Hoguet A, Junk AK, et al. Spectral-domain OCT: helping the clinician diagnose glaucoma: a report by the American Academy of Ophthalmology. *Ophthalmology.* 2018;125(11):1817-1827. doi: 10.1016/j.ophtha.2018.05.008

Schuman JS. Spectral domain optical coherence tomography for glaucoma (an AOS thesis). *Trans Am Ophthalmol Soc.* 2008;106:426-458.

Schuman JS, Hee MR, Puliafito CA, et al. Quantification of nerve fiber layer thickness in normal and glaucomatous eyes using optical coherence tomography. *Arch Ophthalmol.* 1995;113(5):586-596. doi: 10.1001/archopht.1995.01100050054031

Wong JJ, Chen TC, Shen LQ, Pasquale LR. Macular imaging for glaucoma using spectral-domain optical coherence tomography: a review. *Semin Ophthalmol.* 2012;27(5-6):160-166. doi: 10.3109/08820538.2012.712734

Wu H, de Boer JF, Chen TC. Diagnostic capability of spectral-domain optical coherence tomography for glaucoma. *Am J Ophthalmol.* 2012;153(5):815-816. doi: 10.1016/j.ajo.2011.09.032

CHAPTER 22 COMPUTED TOMOGRAPHY AND MAGNETIC RESONANCE IMAGING

Blandford AD, Zhang D, Chundury RV, Perry JD. Dysthyroid optic neuropathy: update on pathogenesis, diagnosis, and management. *Expert Rev Ophthalmol.* 2017;12(2):111-121. doi: 10.1080/17469899.2017.1276444

Cakirer S. MRI findings in Tolosa-Hunt syndrome before and after systemic corticosteroid therapy. *Eur J Radiol.* 2003;45(2):83-90. doi: 10.1016/s0720-048x(02)00012-8

Dutton JJ. *Radiology of the Orbit and Visual Pathways.* Philadelphia, PA: Saunders Elsevier Inc; 2010.

Jarius S, Ruprecht K, Kleiter I, et al. MOG-IgG in NMO and related disorders: a multicenter study of 50 patients. Part 1: frequency, syndrome specificity, influence of disease activity, long-term course, association with AQP4-IgG, and origin. *J Neuroinflammation*. 2016;13(1): 279. doi: 10.1186/s12974-016-0717-1

Johnson MC, Polceni B, Lee AG, Smoker WRK. *Neuroimaging in Ophthalmology*. New York, NY: Oxford University Press; 2011.

Lyrer PA, Brandt T, Metso TM, et al. Clinical import of Horner syndrome in internal carotid and vertebral artery dissection. *Neurology*. 2014;82(18):1653-1659. doi: 10.1212/WNL.0000000000000381

Molitch ME. Nonfunctioning pituitary tumors and pituitary incidentalomas. *Endocrinol Metab Clin North Am*. 2008;37(1):151-171, xi. doi: 10.1016/j.ecl.2007.10.011

Ortiz O, Schochet SS, Kotzan JM, Kostick D. Radiologic-pathologic correlation: meningioma of the optic nerve sheath. *AJNR Am J Neuroradiol*. 1996;17(5):901-906.

Thompson AJ, Banwell BL, Barkhof F, et al. Diagnosis of multiple sclerosis: 2017 revisions of the McDonald criteria. *Lancet Neurol*. 2018;17(2):162-173. doi: 10.1016/S1474-4422(17)30470-2

FINANCIAL DISCLOSURES

Dr. Hasenin Al-khersan has no financial or proprietary interest in the materials presented herein.

Dr. Apostolos Anagnostopoulos has no financial or proprietary interest in the materials presented herein.

Dr. Alessandra Bertolucci has no financial or proprietary interest in the materials presented herein.

Dr. Ying Chen has no financial or proprietary interest in the materials presented herein.

Dr. Sheikh Faheem has no financial or proprietary interest in the materials presented herein.

Dr. Yale Fisher has no financial or proprietary interest in the materials presented herein.

Dr. Daniel Gologorsky has no financial or proprietary interest in the materials presented herein.

Dr. John Hinkle has no financial or proprietary interest in the materials presented herein.

Amy Huang has no financial or proprietary interest in the materials presented herein.

Dr. John W. Latting has no financial or proprietary interest in the materials presented herein.

Dr. Michelle W. Latting has no financial or proprietary interest in the materials presented herein.

Dr. Thomas Lazzarini has no financial or proprietary interest in the materials presented herein.

Dr. Wendy W. Lee has no financial or proprietary interest in the materials presented herein.

Dr. Alexandra E. Levitt has no financial or proprietary interest in the materials presented herein.

Dr. Michael M. Lin has no financial or proprietary interest in the materials presented herein.

Dr. C. Maxwell Medert has no financial or proprietary interest in the materials presented herein.

Dr. Stephen Moster has no financial or proprietary interest in the materials presented herein.

Dr. Nimesh Patel has no financial or proprietary interest in the materials presented herein.

Dr. Ashwinee Ragam has no financial or proprietary interest in the materials presented herein.

Dr. Andrew J. Rong has no financial or proprietary interest in the materials presented herein.

Dr. Richard B. Rosen has personal interest in Opticology and Guardion and is a consultant to OptoVue, Boehringer-Ingelheim, Astellas, Genentech-Roche, NanoRetina, OD-OS, Regeneron, Bayer, Diopsys, Teva, and CellView.

Dr. Oriel Spierer has no financial or proprietary interest in the materials presented herein.

Dr. Ann Q. Tran has no financial or proprietary interest in the materials presented herein.

Dr. Demetrios G. Vavvas has no financial or proprietary interest in the materials presented herein.

Dr. Chris Y. Wu has no financial or proprietary interest in the materials presented herein.

Dr. Cindy X. Zheng has no financial or proprietary interest in the materials presented herein.

INDEX

adaptive optics, 135–147
    chloroquine maculopathy, 140
    chorioretinopathy, 140
    diabetic retinopathy, retinal vein occlusion, 145
    foveal capillary network, avascular zone, 146
    fundus, arteriolar wall structures, 145
    hypertension, 146
    macula-involving retinal detachment, 141
    photopsias, 139
    photoreceptor mosaic, 137
    photoreceptor mosaic defects, 138
    sickle cell retinopathy, 145
    solar retinopathy, 142
    vessel density maps, retinal vein occlusion, 147
angioid streaks, indocyanine green angiography, 96
anterior segment anatomy, orbital ultrasonography, 28–29
anterior segment optical coherence tomography, 51–55
    sclera, layers of, 52–53
    ultrasound biomicroscopy, contrasted, 51–52
Arden ratio, electrophysiology, 169
Artifacts, glaucoma, visual fields, 183
artificial iris implant, diffuse illumination, 33
AS-OCT. *See* anterior segment optical coherence tomography
asteroid hyalosis, vitreous cavity, 155
attenuated inner retinal layers, retinal optical coherence tomography, 115
autofluorescence, fundus, 99–108
    Best disease, 103
    bull's eye maculopathy, 105

central serous retinopathy, 107
dry age-related macular edema, 108
hemorrhagic pigment epithelial detachment, 101
indications, 100–108
interpreting, 100–108
MacTel type 1, 105
multifocal choroiditis, 103
neurosyphilis, 105
optic disc drusen, 104
serpiginous choroiditis, 101
Stargardt's disease, 104
tuberculosis chorioretinitis, 103
uveal melanoma, 102
axial curvature map, 39

B-cell lymphoma, orbital apex, 210
basal cell carcinoma, orbit, nasolacrimal sac, 209
Bell's palsy, reproducibility, external photography, 6
benign ciliary body tumor, 22
bilateral proptosis, reproducibility, external photography, 5–7
biometry for intraocular lens calculations, 61–67
    ultrasound biometry, 62
biomicroscopy, ultrasound, 57–60
branch retinal vein occlusion
    with cystoid macular edema, optical coherence tomography angiography, 126
    fluorescein angiography, 88
canthal region, basal cell carcinoma, 209
carotid artery dissection, carotid canal, with Horner's syndrome, 212

cataract
    nuclear
        dense, optical sectioning, 25
        optical sectioning, 25
    retroillumination, 24
central retinal artery occlusion, global
    hypofluorescence, 87
central retinal venous occlusion, hyperfluorescent
    leakage, fluorescein angiography, 86
chloroquine maculopathy, adaptive optics, 140
chorioretinopathy, adaptive optics, 140
choroidal detachment, 156
choroidal mass, choroid melanoma, 159
choroidal melanoma
    with leaking foci, fluorescein angiography, 90
    with subretinal fluid, retinal optical coherence
        tomography, 115
choroidal neovascular membrane, indocyanine green
    angiography, 95
choroidal neovascularization, indocyanine green
    angiography, 93
choroidal vasculopathy lesion, indocyanine green
    angiography, macular hyperfluorescence, 94
choroideremia, microperimetry, 152
cicatricial ectropion, external photography, 5, 8
ciliary body
    cyst, ultrasound biomicroscopy, 60
    melanoma, ultrasound biomicroscopy, 58
    tumor
        benign, 22
            diffuse illumination, 22
        diffuse illumination, 22
CNV. See choroidal neovascularization
color fundus photo, staphylomatous changes, 79
composition, external photography, 4
computed tomography, 201–212
    neuro-ophthalmology, 201–212
confocal microscopy, 45–49
    endothelial cell layer, 46
    endothelial decompensation, 47
        Fuchs' dystrophy, 47,49
    fungal keratitis with branching filaments, mid-
        corneal stroma, 48
    iridocorneal endothelial syndrome, 48
    microsporidia organisms in corneal stroma, 48
cornea layers, anterior segment optical coherence
    tomography, 52–53
corneal epithelial dendrite, 20
    diffuse cobalt blue light, 20
corneal haze, 26
corneal thickness map, 39
corneal topography, 37–44
    axial curvature map, 39
    corneal thickness map, 39

elevation map, 39
float map, 39
interpretation, 38–44
maps, 38–44
negative Q-values, defined, 38
pentacam axial map
    "bow tie" oblique astigmatism, 41
    pterygium-induced nasal flattening, 41
    tear film abnormalities, 44
pentacam refractive panel, keratoconus, 43
pentacam refractive panel, 40
    after penetrating keratoplasty, 42
placido disc-based imaging, 37–38
Q-value, defined, 38
scanning slit imaging, 38
Scheimpflug imaging, 38
tangential curvature map, 39
corneal ulcer, suture-related, diffuse illumination, 21
crystalline lens dislocation, 157
crystalline stromal dystrophy, optical sectioning, 24
cyclodialysis cleft, ultrasound biomicroscopy, 59
cystoid macular edema, retinal optical coherence
    tomography, 111
cytomegalovirus retinitis, optical coherence
    tomography angiography, 131

dendrite, epithelial, corneal, 20
dense nuclear cataract, optical sectioning, 25
dermatochalasis, lid
    Goldmann visual field, 12, 16
    reproducibility, external photography, 4–5
    static perimetry visual field, 12–13
dermatochalasis repair, external photography, 7–9
Descemet's detachment, ultrasound biomicroscopy,
    59
deviation maps, glaucoma, 177
diabetes without retinopathy, optical coherence
    tomography angiography, 122
diabetic macular edema, retinal optical coherence
    tomography, 111
diabetic retinopathy
    adaptive optics
        retinal vein occlusion, sickle cell
            retinopathy, 145
        sickle cell retinopathy, retinal vein
            occlusion, 145
    fluorescein angiography, 84, 89
    optical coherence tomography angiography, 123
    superficial capillary plexus, optical coherence
        tomography angiography, 122
dislocated intraocular lens, 157
drusen, optical coherence tomography angiography,
    126
dystrophy, stromal, crystalline, optical sectioning, 24

ectropion
  cicatricial, external photography, 5, 8
  lid, reproducibility, external photography, 6
electro-oculogram, vision electrophysiology, 163
electronegative response, vision electrophysiology, 171
electrophysiology, vision, 161–171
  abnormal EOG, Arden ratio, 169
  abnormal mERG, flat responses macula, 168
  electro-oculogram, 163
  electronegative response, 171
  electroretinogram, 162
  flicker stimulus response, 165
  Leber's congenital amaurosis, gene mutation, 166
  multifocal electroretinogram, 162
  normal EOG, 169
  normal mERG, 167
  normal VEP, 170
  scotopic ERG, 165
  visually evoked potential, 163–171
  waveforms, 164
electroretinogram, electrophysiology, 162
elevation map, 39
endothelial cell layer
  confocal microscopy, 46
  Fuchs' disease, confocal microscopy, 49
endothelial decompensation, confocal microscopy, 47
  Fuchs' dystrophy, 47
enophthalmos, CT orbital floor fracture, 208
epiretinal membrane puckering, retinal optical coherence tomography, 114
epithelial dendrite, corneal, 20
epithelial ingrowth, after LASIK, diffuse illumination, 20
erythropsia, adaptive optics, 139
eternal photography, lid ptosis, 9
external photography, 3–9
  cicatricial ectropion, 5, 8
  cicatricial lagophthalmos, 8
  composition, 4
  dermatochalasis repair, 7–9
    lid ptosis, 9
  lagophthalmos, 5, 8
  lid ectropion, reproducibility, 6
  lid nodule, 3–4
  lid ptosis, 9
    dermatochalasis repair, 9
    MRD1, 7–9
    with MRD1, 7–9
    reproducibility, 6
  lighting, 4
  MRD1, lid ptosis, 7–9
  patient positioning, 4–5
  preoperative ptosis, 7–9
  reproducibility, 5–7

Bell's palsy, 6
  bilateral proptosis, 5–7
  lid dermatochalasis, 4–5
  lid ectropion, 6
  lid ptosis, 6
  thyroid eye disease, 5–7
exudative age-related macular degeneration, 76
eyelid. *See* lid

flat responses macula, electrophysiology, 168
flicker stimulus response, electrophysiology, 165
floater map, 39
floaters, 154
"floor effect," glaucoma, 192
fluorescein angiography, 81–92
  blocking, 83
  filling defect, 83
  leakage, 82
  normal, 83
  pooling, 83
  staining, 83
  window defects, 82
focal superior RNFL loss, OCT RNFL analysis display, 186, 190
fornix, symblepharon, diffuse illumination, 25
Fuchs' adenoma, 22
  diffuse illumination, 22
  endothelial cell layer, confocal microscopy, 49
fundus autofluorescence, 99–108
  Best disease, 103
  bull's eye maculopathy, 105
  central serous retinopathy, 107
  dry age-related macular edema, 108
  hemorrhagic pigment epithelial detachment, 101
  indications, 100–108
  interpreting, 100–108
  MacTel type 1, 105
  multifocal choroiditis, 103
  neurosyphilis, 105
  optic disc drusen, 104
  serpiginous choroiditis, 101
  Stargardt's disease, 104
  tuberculosis chorioretinitis, 103
  uveal melanoma, 102
fundus photography, 71–80
  adaptive optics, 144
  color fundus photo, staphylomatous changes, 79
  exudative age-related macular degeneration, 76
  hypertrophy, retinal pigment epithelium, horseshoe tear, 72
  montage fundus photo, choroidal mass, 75
  nonexudative macular degeneration, 76
  peripapillary choroidal melanoma in macula, 75
  red-free fundus photo, calcified drusen, macula, 79

scaphoid preretinal hemorrhage, 77
smartphone fundus photography
    intraocular foreign body, retina, 80
    preretinal hemorrhage, 80
submacular hemorrhage, 78
vitreous detachment, 77
widefield fundus photo
    diabetic retinopathy, 73
    horseshoe tears, 78
    retinal detachment, 75
    retinal venous occlusion, 74
fungal keratitis, 54
    branching filaments, mid-corneal stroma, confocal microscopy, 48

giant cell arteritis, fluorescein angiography, 87
glaucoma, 173–197
    optic nerve, optical coherence tomography angiography, 133
    optical coherence tomography, 185–197
    stimulus size, 176
    visual fields, 175–184
        Goldmann kinetic perimetry, 176
        hill of vision, 175
        multiple fields, 180
        repeat testing, 178–184
        single field analysis, 179
        testing artifacts, 183
        testing strategies, 176–178
            deviation maps, 177
            global indices, 177
            progression analysis, 178
            reliability indices, 176–177
            stimulus size, luminance, testing algorithms, 176
global indices, glaucoma, 177
globe, orbital ultrasonography, 28–29
Goldmann kinetic perimetry, glaucoma, visual fields, 176
Goldmann visual field, upper lid dermatochalasis, 12, 16
granular stromal dystrophy, 53

haze
    corneal, 26
    diffuse, corneal, 26
hemangioma, orbital, 209
Hitachi camera/microscope, 17–18
Horner's syndrome, 212
    carotid artery dissection, carotid canal, 212
hypertrophy, retinal pigment epithelium, horseshoe tear, 72

hypofluorescence, indocyanine green angiography, choroidal tumor, 95
hypofluorescence patterns:, fluorescein angiography, 83

indocyanine green angiography, 93–98
    angioid streaks, 96
    choroidal neovascular membrane, 95
    choroidal neovascularization, 93
    hypofluorescence, choroidal tumor, 95
    macular hotspot, central serous retinopathy, 97
    macular telangiectasia, 94
    polypoidal choroidal vasculopathy, 97
    retinal pigment epithelium, 93
    submacular hemorrhage, 96
    syphilitic placoid lesion, 98
indocyanine green (ICG) angiography, choroidal vasculopathy lesion, macular hyperfluorescence, 94
interfaces, orbital ultrasonography, 27–28
intraocular lens
    capture over iris, diffuse illumination, 23
    dislocated, 157
intraocular lens power calculations, orbital ultrasonography, cataract surgery, 28, 30
iridocorneal endothelial syndrome, confocal microscopy, 48
iris implant
    artificial, diffuse illumination, 33
    diffuse illumination, 33
iris lesion
    diffuse illumination, 22
    pigmented, diffuse illumination, 22
ischemic retina, fluorescein angiography, 91

keratitis, *Acanthamoeba*, diffuse illumination, 21

lagophthalmos, external photography, 5, 8
laser injury, optical coherence tomography angiography, 132
LASIK, 20
    epithelial ingrowth after, diffuse illumination, 20
lattice corneal dystrophy, 55
Leber's congenital amaurosis, gene mutation, electrophysiology, 166
lens power calculations, orbital ultrasonography, cataract surgery, 28, 30
lesion, lid, pigmented, diffuse illumination, 19
lid, ptosis, dermatochalasis repair, external photography, 9
lid dermatochalasis
    Goldmann visual field, 12, 16
    reproducibility, external photography, 4–5
    static perimetry visual field, 12–13

lid lesion, pigmented, diffuse illumination, 19

lid ptosis

external photography, 9

with MRD1, 7–9

photography, 9

reproducibility, external photography, 6

static perimetry visual field, 12, 14–15

lighting, external photography, 4

luminance, defined, microperimetry, 150

macroadenoma, pituitary, 213

macula-involving retinal detachment, adaptive optics, 141

macular degeneration, choroidal neovascular membrane, fluorescein angiography, 90

macular degeneration with drusen, retinal optical coherence tomography, 112

macular degeneration with hemorrhage, edema, retinal optical coherence tomography, 112

macular hole with hyaloid separation, cystoid hydration, OCT, 113

macular hotspot, indocyanine green angiography, central serous retinopathy, 97

macular retinal ganglion cell layer, optical coherence tomography, glaucoma, 191

macular telangiectasia

indocyanine green angiography, 94

optical coherence tomography angiography, 130

magnetic resonance imaging, 201–212

neuro-ophthalmology, 201–212

masticator space, venous malformation, 212

meningioma, optic nerve sheath, 213

microperimetry, 149–152

choroideremia, 152

luminance, defined, 150

retinal microperimetry, indications, 149–150

retinal microperimetry, 151

retinal perimetry, interpreting, 150–152

sensitivity, defined, 150

terms, 150–152

microsporidia organisms in corneal stroma, confocal microscopy, 48

montage fundus photo, choroidal mass, 75

MRD1, lid ptosis, external photography, 7–9

mucocele, sinus, 212

multifocal electroretinogram, electrophysiology, 162

multiple fields, glaucoma, visual fields, 180

multiple sclerosis, periventricular demyelinating lesions, optic neuritis, 211

muscle belly enlargement, thyroid eye disease, without muscle insertion, 31, 33

nasal bulbar conjunctival pigmented lesion, diffuse illumination, 19

nasolacrimal sac, orbit, basal cell carcinoma, 209

negative Q-values, defined, 38

neovascularization of disc, fluorescein angiography, diabetic retinopathy, 91

neuro-ophthalmology, 199–212

computed tomography, 201–212

magnetic resonance imaging, 201–212

nodule, lid, external photography, 3–4

nonexudative age-related macular degeneration, window defect, fluorescein angiography, 85

nonexudative macular degeneration, 76

nuclear cataract

dense, optical sectioning, 25

optical sectioning, 25

oculoplastics, 1–33

external photography, 3–9

cicatricial ectropion, 5, 8

cicatricial lagophthalmos, 8

composition, 4

dermatochalasis repair, 7–9

lid nodule, 3–4

lid ptosis, 9

with MRD1, 7–9

patient positioning, 4–5

reproducibility, 5–7

Bell's palsy, 6

bilateral proptosis, 5–7

lid dermatochalasis, 4–5

lid ectropion, 6

lid ptosis, 6

orbital ultrasonography, 27–33

anterior segment anatomy, 28–29

globe, 28–29

interfaces, 27–28

intraocular lens power calculations, cataract surgery, 28, 30

optic nerve on ultrasound, 28, 30

orbital hemangioma, 31–32

orbital lymphangioma, fluid-filled cysts, 31–32

orbital lymphoma, 28, 30

retinal detachment, 27–29

Rosai-Dorfman disease, 29, 31

ptosis visual fields, 11–16

Goldmann visual field, upper lid dermatochalasis, 12, 16

static perimetry visual field

lid dermatochalasis, 12–13

patient with lid ptosis, 12, 14–15

slit lamp photography, 17–26

cataract, posterior, retroillumination, 24

diffuse cobalt blue light, corneal epithelial dendrite, 20

diffuse corneal haze, 26

diffuse illumination

artificial iris implant, 33

epithelial ingrowth after LASIK, 20

Fuchs' adenoma, 22
intraocular lens, capture over iris, 23
pigmented iris lesion, 22
suspected case of *Acanthamoeba*
    keratitis, 21
suture-related corneal ulcer, 21
symblepharon in inferior fornix, 25
diffuse illumination, pigmented eyelid
    lesion, 19
Hitachi camera/microscope, 17–18
nasal bulbar conjunctival pigmented lesion,
    diffuse illumination, 19
optical sectioning
    crystalline stromal dystrophy, 24
    dense nuclear cataract, 25
    superotemporal scleral melt, uveal
        protrusion, 19
sclerotic scatter examination, 25
optic disc neovascularization, diabetic retinopathy,
    optical coherence tomography angiography, 123
optic nerve
    glaucoma, optical coherence tomography
        angiography, 133
    orbital ultrasonography, 28, 30
optic nerve head, optical coherence tomography,
    glaucoma, 191
optic nerve sheath, meningioma, 213
optic neuritis, periventricular demyelinating lesions,
    multiple sclerosis, 211
optical coherence tomography
    glaucoma, 185–197
        "floor effect" in glaucoma, 192
        macular retinal ganglion cell layer, 191
        OCT RNFL analysis, RNFL thinning,
            186, 189
        OCT RNFL analysis display
            focal superior RNFL loss, 186, 190
            no glaucomatous damage, 186–187
            signal loss artifact, 186, 188
        OCT RNFL progression analysis, RNFL
            loss, 195–197
        optic nerve head, 191
        pitfalls, 186–191
        progression analysis, 191–195
        retina, 69–72
        retinal nerve fiber layer, 186–191
    retina, 109–117
        attenuated inner retinal layers, after central
            retinal artery occlusion, 115
        choroidal melanoma with subretinal fluid,
            115
        cystoid macular edema, 111
        diabetic macular edema, diabetic
            retinopathy, 111
        epiretinal membrane puckering macular
            surface, 114

macular degeneration with drusen, 112
macular degeneration with hemorrhage,
    edema, 112
macular hole with hyaloid separation,
    cystoid hydration, 113
normal retina, 110
signal hyper-transmission, 115
staphylomatous eye, atrophy, 113
vitreomacular traction, thickened hyaloid
    face, 114
X-linked retinoschisis, schisis cavities, 116
optical coherence tomography angiography, 119–134
    branch retinal vein occlusion, with cystoid
        macular edema, 126
    diabetes without retinopathy, 122
    diabetic retinopathy, 123
    drusen, 126
    optic disc neovascularization, diabetic
        retinopathy, 123
    polypoidal choroidal vasculopathy, 125
    retinal angiomatous proliferation, 128
    retinal vascular layers, 121
    subretinal CNV, 127
    superficial capillary plexus, diabetic retinopathy,
        122
optical sectioning
    crystalline stromal dystrophy, 24
    dense nuclear cataract, 25
    rheumatoid arthritis, 19
    superotemporal scleral melt, uveal protrusion,
        19
        rheumatoid arthritis, 19
    uveal protrusion
        rheumatoid arthritis, 19
        superotemporal scleral melt, rheumatoid
            arthritis, 19
orbit
    basal cell carcinoma, nasolacrimal sac, 209
    orbital ultrasonography, 28–29
    subperiosteal abscess, 207
    temporal fossa, masticator space, venous
        malformation, 212
orbital apex, B-cell lymphoma, 210
orbital floor fracture, enophthalmos, 208
orbital hemangioma, 209
    orbital ultrasonography, 31–32
orbital lymphangioma, orbital ultrasonography, fluid-
    filled cysts, 31–32
orbital lymphoma, orbital ultrasonography, 28, 30
orbital ultrasonography, 27–33
    anterior segment anatomy, 28–29
    globe, 28–29
    interfaces, 27–28
    intraocular lens power calculations, cataract
        surgery, 28, 30
    optic nerve on ultrasound, 28, 30

orbit, 28–29
orbital hemangioma, 31–32
orbital lymphangioma, fluid-filled cysts, 31–32
orbital lymphoma, 28, 30
retinal detachment, 27–29
Rosai-Dorfman disease, 29, 31
Tenon's space, scleritis, 31, 33
thyroid eye disease, muscle belly enlargement,
    31–33

papilledema, optical coherence tomography
    angiography, 134
patient positioning, external photography, 4–5
pentacam axial map
    "bow tie" oblique astigmatism, 41
    pterygium-induced nasal flattening, 41
    tear film abnormalities, 44
pentacam refractive panel, 40
    after penetrating keratoplasty, 42
pentacam refractive panel, keratoconus, 43
peripapillary choroidal melanoma in macula, 75
periventricular demyelinating lesions, optic neuritis,
    multiple sclerosis, 211
phakic eyes, biometry for intraocular lens
    calculations, 64, 67
photopsias, adaptive optics, 139
photoreceptor mosaic, adaptive optics, 137
photoreceptor mosaic defects, adaptive optics, 138
pigmented eyelid lesion, diffuse illumination, 19
pigmented iris lesion, diffuse illumination, 22
pituitary macroadenoma, 213
placido disc-based imaging, 37–38
plateau iris, ultrasound biomicroscopy, 58
polypoidal choroidal vasculopathy
    indocyanine green angiography, 97
    optical coherence tomography angiography, 125
preoperative, external photography, ptosis, 7–9
preoperative ptosis, external photography, 7–9
progression analysis
    glaucoma, 178
    optical coherence tomography, glaucoma,
        191–195
proptosis, bilateral, reproducibility, external
    photography, 5–7
pseudophakic eye, ultrasound biomicroscopy, 60
pterygium, slit lamp photo, 53
ptosis
    lid
        dermatochalasis repair, external
            photography, 9
        external photography, with MRD1, 7–9
        MRD1, external photography, 7–9
        photography, 9
        reproducibility, external photography, 6
        static perimetry visual field, 12, 14–15
    preoperative, external photography, 7–9

ptosis visual fields, 11–16
    Goldmann visual field, upper lid
        dermatochalasis, 12, 16
    static perimetry visual field
        lid dermatochalasis, 12–13
        patient with lid ptosis, 12, 14–15

Q-value, defined, 38

red-free fundus photo, calcified drusen, macula, 79
reliability indices, glaucoma, 176–177
reproducibility
    Bell's palsy, external photography, 6
    bilateral proptosis, external photography, 5–7
    external photography, 5–7
    lid dermatochalasis, external photography, 4–5
    lid ectropion, external photography, 6
retina, 69–171
retinal angiomatous proliferation, optical coherence
    tomography angiography, 128
retinal detachment, 159
    orbital ultrasonography, 27–29
retinal flap tear, 158
retinal microperimetry, microperimetry, indications,
    149–150
retinal microperimetry, microperimetry, 151
retinal necrosis
    opacification/hemorrhage, optical coherence
        tomography angiography, 129
    optical coherence tomography angiography, 129
retinal nerve fiber layer, optical coherence
    tomography, glaucoma, 186–191
retinal optical coherence tomography, 109–117
    attenuated inner retinal layers, after central
        retinal artery occlusion, 115
    choroidal melanoma with subretinal fluid, 115
    cystoid macular edema, 111
    diabetic macular edema, diabetic retinopathy,
        111
    epiretinal membrane puckering macular surface,
        114
    macular degeneration with drusen, 112
    macular degeneration with hemorrhage, edema,
        112
    macular hole with hyaloid separation, cystoid
        hydration, 113
    normal retina, 110
    signal hyper-transmission, 115
    staphylomatous eye, atrophy, 113
    vitreomacular traction, thickened hyaloid face,
        114
    X-linked retinoschisis, schisis cavities, 116
retinal perimetry, interpreting, microperimetry,
    150–152
retinal pigment epithelium, indocyanine green
    angiography, 93

retinal ultrasonography, 153–159
  anomalous optic nerve evaluation, 157
  asteroid hyalosis, vitreous cavity, 155
  choroidal detachment, 156
  choroidal mass, choroid melanoma, 159
  crystalline lens dislocation, 157
  excavation at posterior pole, staphyloma, 159
  floaters, 154
  intraocular lens, dislocated, 157
  orbit, 154
  retinal flap tear, 158
  total retinal detachment, 159
  vitreous detachment, 156
    with floaters, 155
retinal vascular layers, optical coherence tomography angiography, 121
retinopathy, fluorescein angiography, 92
rheumatoid arthritis, optical sectioning, 19
Rosai-Dorfman disease, orbital ultrasonography, 29, 31
RPE. *See* retinal pigment epithelium

Salzmann nodular degeneration, 55
scanning slit imaging, 38
scaphoid preretinal hemorrhage, 77
Scheimpflug imaging, 38
schwannoma, orbit, soft tissue window, 208
scleritis, Tenon's space, orbital ultrasonography, 31, 33
sclerotic scatter examination, 25
sea fan neovascularization with temporal leakage, sickle-cell retinopathy, fluorescein angiography, 86
sensitivity, defined, microperimetry, 150
sickle-cell retinopathy, sea fan neovascularization with temporal leakage, fluorescein angiography, 86
signal hyper-transmission, retinal optical coherence tomography, 115
signal loss artifact, OCT RNFL analysis display, 186, 188
single field analysis, glaucoma, visual fields, 179
sinus mucocele, 212
slit lamp photography, 17–26
  cataract, posterior, retroillumination, 24
  corneal epithelial dendrite, diffuse cobalt blue light, 20
  corneal haze, 26
  crystalline stromal dystrophy, optical sectioning, 24
  dense nuclear cataract, optical sectioning, 25
  diffuse cobalt blue light, corneal epithelial dendrite, 20
  diffuse corneal haze, 26
  diffuse illumination

    artificial iris implant, 33
    ciliary body tumor, 22
    epithelial ingrowth after LASIK, 20
    Fuchs' adenoma, 22
    intraocular lens, capture over iris, 23
    iris implant, 33
    iris lesion, 22
    pigmented iris lesion, 22
    suspected case of *Acanthamoeba* keratitis, 21
    suture-related corneal ulcer, 21
    symblepharon in inferior fornix, 25
  diffuse illumination, pigmented eyelid lesion, 19
  epithelial ingrowth after LASIK, diffuse illumination, 20
  Hitachi camera/microscope, 17–18
  nasal bulbar conjunctival pigmented lesion, diffuse illumination, 19
  optical sectioning
    crystalline stromal dystrophy, 24
    dense nuclear cataract, 25
    rheumatoid arthritis, 19
    superotemporal scleral melt, uveal protrusion, 19
    uveal protrusion
      rheumatoid arthritis, 19
      superotemporal scleral melt, rheumatoid arthritis, 19
  pigmented eyelid lesion, diffuse illumination, 19
  sclerotic scatter examination, 25
  suture-related corneal ulcer, diffuse illumination, 21
  symblepharon, inferior fornix, diffuse illumination, 25
smartphone fundus photography
  intraocular foreign body, retina, 80
  preretinal hemorrhage, 80
solar retinopathy, Amsler grid, adaptive optics, 142
sphenoid, greater wing fibrous dysplasia, 206
squamous neoplasia, 53–54
staphyloma, excavation at posterior pole, 159
staphylomatous eye, retinal optical coherence tomography, atrophy, 113
static perimetry visual field
  lid dermatochalasis, 12–13
  lid ptosis, 12, 14–15
stromal dystrophy, crystalline, optical sectioning, 24
submacular hemorrhage, 78
  indocyanine green angiography, 96
subcapsular cataracts, biometry for intraocular lens calculations, 66
superior branch retinal artery occlusion, fluorescein angiography, 87
superotemporal scleral melt, uveal protrusion, optical sectioning, 19

suture-related corneal ulcer, diffuse illumination, 21

symblepharon, inferior fornix, diffuse illumination, 25

syphilitic placoid lesion, indocyanine green angiography, 98

tangential curvature map, 39

TED. *See* thyroid eye disease

temporal fossa, masticator space, venous malformation, 212

Tenon's space, orbital ultrasonography, scleritis, 31, 33

testing artifacts, glaucoma, visual fields, 183

testing strategies, glaucoma, 176–178
    deviation maps, 177
    global indices, 177
    reliability indices, 176–177
    stimulus size, 176

thyroid eye disease
    compressive optic neuropathy, 207
    orbital ultrasonography, muscle belly enlargement, 31–33
    reproducibility, external photography, 5–7

ultrasonography, retinal, 153–159
    asteroid hyalosis, vitreous cavity, 155
    choroidal mass, choroid melanoma, 159
    crystalline lens dislocation, 157
    excavation at posterior pole, staphyloma, 159
    intraocular lens, dislocated, 157
    retinal flap tear, ultrasound, 158
    total retinal detachment, ultrasound, 159
    ultrasonography, anomalous optic nerve evaluation, 157
    ultrasound, 154
        choroidal detachment, 156
        floaters, 154
        orbit, 154
        vitreous detachment, 156
            with floaters, 155

ultrasound biomicroscopy, 57–60
    anterior segment optical coherence tomography, contrasted, 51–52
    contrasted, anterior segment optical coherence tomography, 51–52

uveal protrusion, rheumatoid arthritis, optical sectioning, 19

venous malformation, orbit, temporal fossa, masticator space, 212

vision electrophysiology, 161–171
    abnormal EOG, Arden ratio, 169
    abnormal mERG, flat responses macula, 168
    electro-oculogram, 163
    electronegative response, 161
    electroretinogram, 162
    flicker stimulus response, 165
    Leber's congenital amaurosis, gene mutation, 166
    multifocal electroretinogram, 162
    normal EOG, 169
    normal mERG, 167
    normal VEP, 170
    scotopic ERG, 165
    visually evoked potential, 163–171
    waveforms, 164

visually evoked potential, vision electrophysiology, 163–171

vitreomacular traction, retinal optical coherence tomography, thickened hyaloid face, 114

vitreous cavity, scintillating hyperechoic debris, 155

vitreous detachment, 77, 156
    with floaters, 155

waveforms, electrophysiology, 164

widefield fundus photo
    diabetic retinopathy, 73
    horseshoe tears, 78
    retinal detachment, 75
    retinal venous occlusion, 74

window defect, fluorescein angiography, "bull's eye" maculopathy, retinal pigment epitheliopathy, 89

X-linked retinoschisis, retinal optical coherence tomography, schisis cavities, 116

Printed in the United States
by Baker & Taylor Publisher Services